BODY
BY
GILDA

BODY BY GILDA

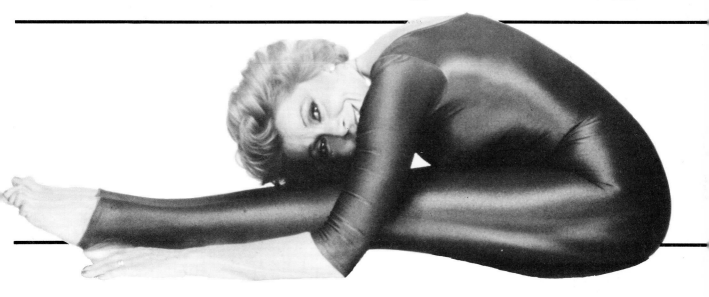

BY GILDA MARX

REDESIGN EVERY LINE

G. P. PUTNAM'S SONS   NEW YORK

Library of Congress Cataloging in Publication Data

Marx, Gilda.
  Body by Gilda.

  1. Reducing exercises.   2. Exercise for women.
I. Title.
RA781.6.M37   1984   646.7′5   83-23007
ISBN 0-399-12918-9

Printed in the United States of America

To my dear mother, Ruth,
who has always had the energy for me—
and the rest of her family.

ACKNOWLEDGMENTS

There are certain people whose help and encouragement were invaluable and I would like to take this opportunity to thank them individually. First and foremost is my husband, Robert Marx, whose immeasurable talent, sense of humor and ever-constant support and love helped to make this book a reality. Jason Thomas for his contribution and assistance. I also wish to thank my Board of Medical Advisors for contributing their specialized knowledge and expertise: Robert Forster, Registered Physical Therapist, a dedicated professional in the field of sports medicine, who has done extensive research with the Body Design by Gilda program in aerobic injury prevention; Dr. Daniel Silver, Orthopedic Surgeon; Dr. Morry Waksberg, Ophthalmic Surgeon; Dr. Gary Tearston, Reconstructive Surgeon; and Dr. Mark Saginor, Internist. And for going beyond the call of duty, Debi Hodgen, manager of the Body Design by Gilda Century City Studio, and my entire Body Design by Gilda staff. I greatly appreciate their devotion and assistance.

And finally, the professionals whose combined talents resulted in a book that is a work of art: Scott Orazem, photographer; Marie Pierre Pappallardo, hair; and Michelle Van Der Hule, makeup.

CONTENTS

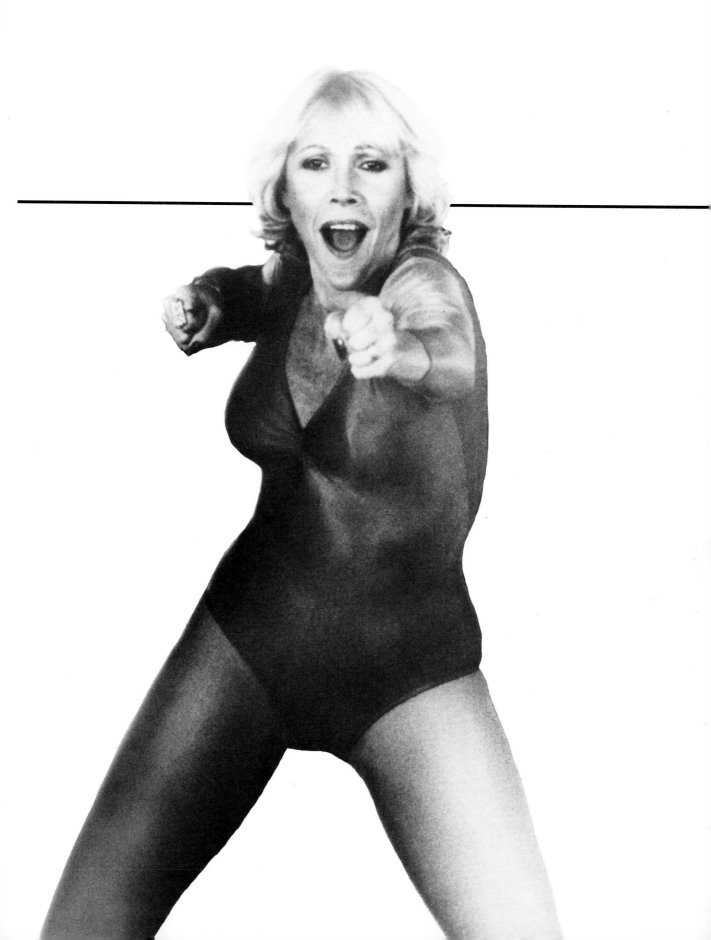

BODY
BY
GILDA

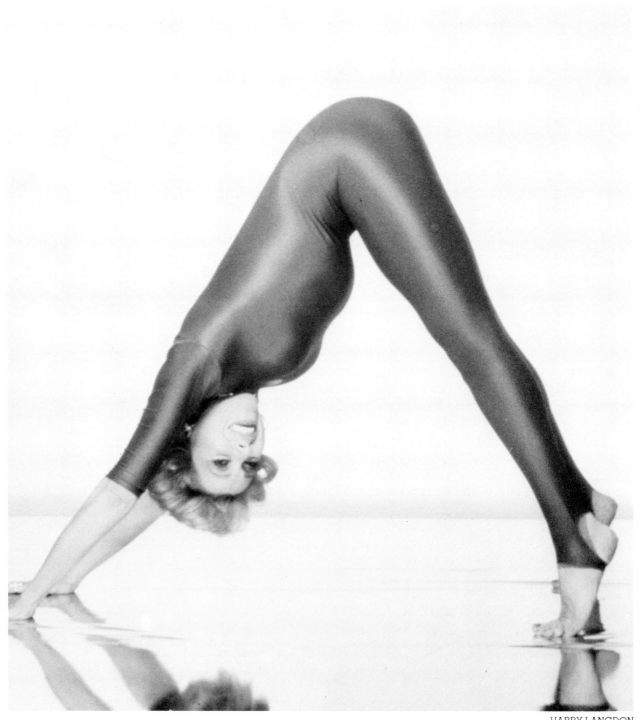

14 | BODY BY GILDA

CHAPTER 1

YOU CAN DO IT!

*Most powerful is he who
has himself in his power.*
—LUCIUS ANNAEUS SENECA

You can do it!

You can have it all. You can awaken in the morning filled with energy. You can have great health. You can look in the mirror a hundred times a day and see a person with the sculptured, well-shaped body you have always wanted. And that energy-packed, healthy, sleek person will be you.

But . . .

You have to be the one who makes this happen. Don't worry. You won't be alone. As you progress through the Body Design by Gilda program, I will be there to help, just as my training has helped more than 250,000 people during the last twenty years.

While a perfectly proportioned body is a fortunate gift of heredity and nature, many people who think they have awkward and lumpy bodies do have hope. Often a fine body has been hidden under layers of excess flesh or disguised by poor posture. A healthy and trim body is a gift only you can give to yourself.

You can't simply write a check to buy health and sleekness. We are all equal when it comes to exercise. A rich person cannot hire someone to do surrogate push-ups or leg lifts. If you want something badly enough, you have to work for it. Everything takes work.

Barbra Streisand is an example.

If anything, Barbra has to watch to keep her body in shape more than someone who is not in the public eye. People notice immediately when Barbra adds a few pounds. This puts even more pressure on her. When Barbra first walked into my penthouse exercise studio overlooking Beverly Hills, she seemed totally unaware of her fitness potential. Certainly she is a secure person as far as her voice and acting ability are concerned, but fitness-wise and coordination-wise, Barbra thought she was a klutz.

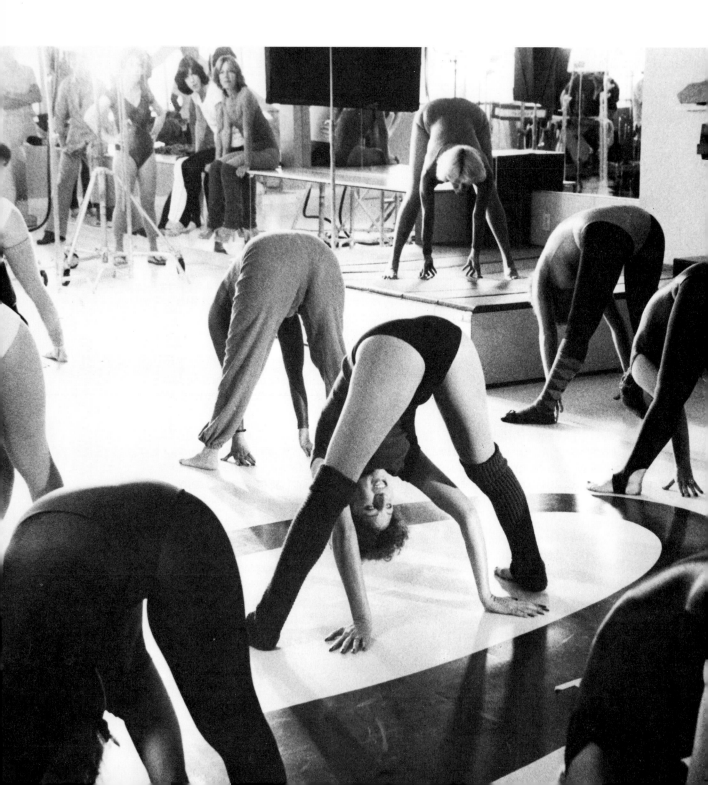

Actually Barbra Streisand is not a klutz.

She worried that she lacked coordination. She was totally unaware that she had great legs and a most remarkable derriere. It was a revelation for her to discover that she could be coordinated, that she did look graceful when she was moving, and that she had a body that did not have to be hidden in layers of carefully designed costumes.

Barbra took fitness seriously. She made the Body Design by Gilda program her workout.

Barbra Streisand had to sweat and stretch and, yes, ache for many hours to achieve the new shape and the added energy that she has today. No one did it for her. She could not use a stand-in here.

The Body Design by Gilda program is not an instant cure for a drooping something or a flabby whatever. The program does not include any miracle secrets. I will not be suggesting that you make the mango a basic staple of your diet.

In fact, I am against dieting!

Now, don't go getting your hopes aroused. Just because I disapprove of dieting does not mean that you should lay in a supply of French vanilla ice cream and hot fudge. I don't believe in fad diets. I do believe in proper nutrition. I do believe in the activity-versus-calories syndrome. It's really just common sense. You eat the foods that are needed to satisfy your body and keep it in good health.

The Body Design by Gilda program is the result of twenty years of common sense. Common sense about the advantage of proper exercise. Common sense about what and how much you eat. Common sense about your own body. Instead of being a fad, the Body Design by Gilda program is a way of life that will result in a healthier, happier, and better-looking you.

I have witnessed so many success stories in my two decades of operating some of the finest exercise studios in the world. I have seen people with extreme problems transform themselves into what they always wanted to be. While physical reshaping is an important part of the Body Design by Gilda program, it is only part of the program. The other part, often more satisfying in the end, is the emotional improvement. As the inches or pounds start to reshape and disappear, an exuberant bounce comes into your step. Better still, that energy, the energy of success, changes you even more on the inside than the stretches, sit-ups, and jumping jacks have altered your exterior. This is the result of the I-can-do-it philosophy. You will have more ambition. You will be proud of your new-found self-discipline. You will know that you can succeed. This psychological high appears with the first few hints of success. Maybe the waist is an inch thinner. Maybe the thighs seem a little smoother. The smallest external improvement can launch a whole new self-assured attitude. It's a wonderful feeling, this natural high. Sometimes this happens during the very first workout, when you feel that first rush of new energy. This is a first-rate feeling. It is at this moment that your life changes. The best part is that this high can last the rest of your life.

My program is meant to be a total lifetime philosophy that couples a new attitude toward the importance of food in your life with a daily fitness plan that exercises and interrelates every muscle of your body. It creates mental and physical harmony. As each muscle and tendon gains tone, strength and firmness, the whole body improves. The program extends to every cubic inch of the body. It is not limited to specialized areas. The improvement is everywhere.

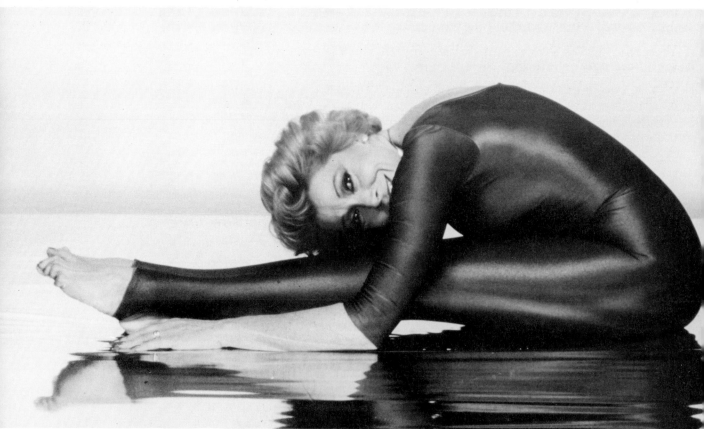

HARRY LANGDON

The final result: a whole new you.

Creating that "new you" requires that a lot of probing questions be asked of the "old you." Even more difficult than asking yourself what is to blame for that lack of energy, those extra pounds, and those misplaced inches, is to change the way you think and live so that, once corrected, these problems stay corrected.

For instance: say you have more inches than you want around your middle. Getting rid of a spare tire is not that difficult. Exercise to tighten the muscles. Cut back on the amount of calories consumed in a day. Correct bad posture. Suddenly that tire is deflated. All finished—right?

Wrong!

That spare tire is far from gone. Instead, it is hiding inside that svelte body, waiting for those newly strengthened muscles to sag from disuse, waiting for a few extra helpings of potatoes, just waiting to reappear. Your psychological habits caused that tire to form in the first place. Those habits must go. Those habits must be replaced with new habits if that tire is to be banished forever.

You are the person who must sit down and analyze what is going on with your life, what will never really change, and decide to readapt your reactions to these forces. You can't always change your environment, but you can change the way you respond to that environment.

- Stop "harming" yourself by over-eating.
- Stop "harming" yourself by over-fatiguing.
- Stop "harming" yourself by over-drinking.
- Stop "harming" yourself by being with negative people who make you feel uncomfortable.

So many people seem to respond to life's frustrations and hurts by doing something that hurts them even more than any negative outside influences. That just isn't common sense. Common sense is changing the negative circumstances right now, right this minute. Common sense is getting a hold of yourself. You are the one who can make the change. Nobody else can do it for you.

Picture yourself the way you really want to be. Think about firming and reshaping that body. Think pride. Think of the better health you will have. Think of the glow that will radiate from you. Think of yourself as sleek. Think of yourself as a happy person. Start to change yourself, now, this second. It will be an inner change, your new mental attitude, that will ultimately rearrange that outer flesh and muscle.

You are the one who has permitted yourself to become out-of-shape and out-of-energy. You are the one who must change yourself.

A Gilda Rule: Stop Being Your Own Enemy.

- Just because you might not have achieved everything you had hoped for in your career, don't reward yourself with extra helpings of desserts. Reward your body with exercise.
- Just because your children might not be exactly what you had hoped, don't sit around the house worrying. Make yourself exactly what *you* want to be.
- Just because you are lonely, don't make your best friend the refrigerator.
- Just because the day was a bummer, don't block out the world by sitting in front of the television, surrounded by food and inactivity.

Start to think, be aware of what you are doing to yourself. Crises are always going to be part of life. Crises should be overcome, not used as excuses. People have never solved life's problems by making themselves less healthy and more unattractive. But for some reason, this is exactly what people do.

People have to stop blaming their inability to be disciplined on the problems of hour-to-hour, day-to-day and month-to-month living.

The Body Design by Gilda program helps you to change your inner attitude toward yourself. Then, through a program that unites good nutrition with a carefully planned group of daily exercises, your new inner self resculptures your old outer self.

The Body Design by Gilda program is definitely anti-fad. This program is against fad diets with their usual, predictable short-term results. The Body Design by Gilda program is also against fad exercising—and the fad exerciser. This is the person who finds some extra padding forming and races off to exercise three times a day. This binger can be found limping around a jogging track, huffing to the point of exhaustion at an exercise studio or gym, and waiting in line at the drugstore to purchase a large-sized bottle of Absorbine Jr.

The Body by Gilda program is a circular process: the body needs—it must have—a proper combination of nutrition *and* regular DAILY exercise to thrive. What hurts the body is that day when you decide to skip exercising (just this once) and all those now unneeded calories start to accumulate. And we all know what happens to unneeded calories—they turn to fat. Unfortunately, it is that all-too-human urge to avoid exertion, either of the mental or physical variety. This is where ruination begins. This is the start of the fitness battle. *A Gilda Rule: When You Skip Exercising, Even Once, Cut the Amount of Food Consumed.* This is a start to fitness and health awareness.

Instead of avoiding exercise, you should be training yourself to seek out exercise opportunities. A stairway is actually a chance to burn a few unwanted and unneeded calories while reshaping the calf muscles. A donut shop is not a place of glazed rewards for a lonesome stomach, but a motivation to spur feet to move quickly away while you straighten your back and breathe deeply, filling your system with low calorie-high energy air.

Too often, fad-binging is followed by guilt. Either aching muscles or a too-full stomach reminds you that you have overpushed or overstuffed your body, that body that you intended to make fit. You become depressed. You need something to cheer you. Maybe a hot fudge sundae. Maybe four hours of sitting through a double feature with a tub of extra-buttered popcorn for companionship. This is the emotional cycle that must be broken if you are going to reshape yourself for the rest of your life.

You must break that pattern. How? You break that pattern when you don't use food or laziness as a reward to make up for the unfairness of life. You break that pattern by saying, "I don't need that hot fudge sundae. I am proud of myself because I can resist that hot fudge sundae. I have just made myself a stronger person because I was capable of refusing something that would have prevented me from reaching my goal."

This is the championship, pattern-breaking attitude.

All this philosophy is a simplistic look at the solution to a very complex—and very human—psychological problem. *A Gilda Rule: When You Are Down, Don't Do Things That Will Result in Still More Damage. Instead, Turn Toward Doing Things to Improve Yourself So That You Will Have the Pride and Strength to Overcome Those Problems.* Exchange all that negative energy for positive energy.

Again! If you can escape from being governed by your emotions, at the same time accepting what is happening to you even if what is happening is totally unpleasant, and go forward with your life—then you are WINNING!

CHAPTER 2
YOU ARE NOT ALONE!

If life had a second edition,
how I would correct the proofs.
—PERCY BYSSHE SHELLEY

Yes, I have been there.

I was fat. It still hurts me to say that word, "FAT!!!" Just a simple three-letter word that has caused so much emotional pain for so many millions of people. Fat hurts in so many ways.

I have been through the trauma of being a fat girl. I remember the cruel remarks from my classmates. I know how it is to be ugly and unaccepted. This happened in my childhood and teenage years. I was born in Pittsburgh. My family was middle class, large (four children), and very, very happy. My weight problem was not built on misery, but on affection.

The very best time of the day for my family was when we all gathered together at the dinner table, talking and joking and showing interest in each other. It was only natural that we all tried to prolong those dinners with extra helpings of everything.

Such food! Stuffed veal breasts. Roast brisket of beef swimming in thick juices. Delicious chicken soup. Roasted chicken. And mashed potatoes. My mother was such a wonderful cook and had an appreciative family waiting for every calorie-packed morsel. But who knew about calories or cared about them then? Calories didn't matter. Rich gravies did. Mother loved to cook and loved to see us eat. It was home, it was secure. It was love.

I loved to eat.

But while all that food and love seemed so wonderful at home, where a few pounds always seemed to go unnoticed, the outside world was not so kind to me.

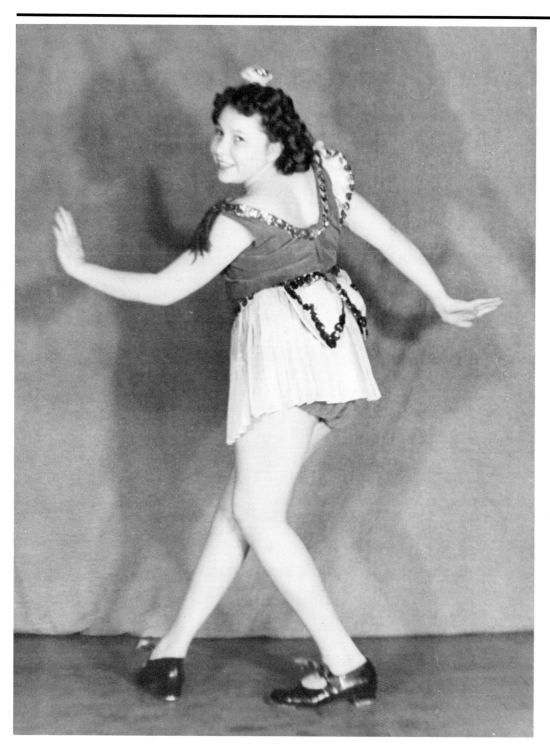

Out there I was "Hey, Fattie!"

Childhood ridicule seems to scar for a lifetime. Those words are still painful. Childhood habits mold the adult.

For me, everything seemed confused. On one side, food was equated with affection, security and good family times. On the other, food resulted in cruel insults, ugly clothes from the chubby (a horrible word) area of Kaufman's Department Store, and disapproving stares on the street. Fat wasn't comfortable. Fat wasn't pretty. Fat wasn't something I wanted to be. Yet the best place in the world was my home, a home filled with love and food. Eating became a refuge from the outside world.

Fortunately, I loved physical activity. I wanted to dance. I didn't care if I was a fat dancer (well, maybe I did care, but I refused to let my weight keep me from dancing). I was gifted with energy. But even all that energy was not enough to burn away all the calories I was consuming. I was simply eating too much.

There was a turning point.

It was comfortable and exciting for me to get up in front of people and talk and sing and dance. I took dance lessons as a small child. Every six months that dance studio had a show. When I first walked on the stage, the audience immediately reacted to my weight and my round little body. They gawked and wondered what that little fat girl was going to do out there in front of the footlights.

"Look at that fat little girl," someone said loudly as I tapped onto the stage with my chubette torso (a 34-inch waist at age eight) propped on surprisingly slender legs.

I kept dancing.

"Boy, she's good," was the next comment. At that moment, pride started to replace insecurity, and I danced all the harder.

"She's great," was the last comment I heard before the noise of the audience mixed into a thunder of approval. By the end of my number, people were standing and applauding fat little me. Applause is wonderful. This moment changed my life.

Maybe I didn't realize it then, but I had just had my first taste of inner success, inner resolve, and inner pride. I kept dancing . . . exercising . . . because I made myself feel proud. I did it alone. It was the embryo of the philosophy behind the Body Design by Gilda program.

Thank God for the man who said, "She's great." We all need support. That is what I try to give the people who follow my program. Support. You are great just for trying. You can be greater still. We can have it all. That moment has been the key to success for me. We all need those moments when we are attracting applause and approval. I know that I will never forget my first applause.

Even though I was no longer fat at the age of sixteen, I was in my middle thirties before I started believing that I was truly a thin person. Somehow, inside, I always felt fat. Bitter memories do linger.

I haven't been fat for a long time (don't ask how long). I will never be fat again because I have changed my attitude toward fattening foods. I discovered the importance of exercise. I changed my attitude toward myself.

A part of my life is a carefully programmed daily calisthenic and aerobics session that includes a lot of stretching. Every day I work out. Every day I watch the foods that I put into that body I worked so hard to create.

I live my program and because of that program and my life, hundreds of thousands of people now know how to stay permanently fit, healthy and happy.

The Body Design by Gilda exercise routine is a complete physical workout. No muscle in the body is neglected. The important difference between my program and all the other programs is that my exercises are planned to develop every muscle in the body in relationship to all the other muscles in the body. For instance: my leg exercises work one part of the leg . . . then another . . . then another in a carefully planned sequence. The result: not only a shaplier leg but a stronger, more powerful leg.

Being physically fit involves strength, firmness and muscle tone, flexibility and suppleness, stamina and endurance as well as the ability to feel relaxed, physically untensed and happy. Sports are fine, but seldom is a single sport enough to make a person totally fit. Few of the athletes you see on television are completely in shape. Football players, for instance, often have hugely developed torsos, massive arms and strong legs, but need aerobics to improve the cardiovascular system. Most sports cover some, but not all, of the fitness bases. Some of the muscle groups are ignored.

The Body Design by Gilda program covers everything.

It has shown hundreds of thousands of overweight, out-of-shape people how to find mental and physical fitness. The gain in flexibility and muscular strength, after a few weeks of the program, makes you better prepared to handle the demands of everyday life. Simple tasks, like carrying packages, become easier. Climbing stairs becomes an exercise instead of a chore. This program is not just a means to a better-looking you, it is a means to a better quality of life.

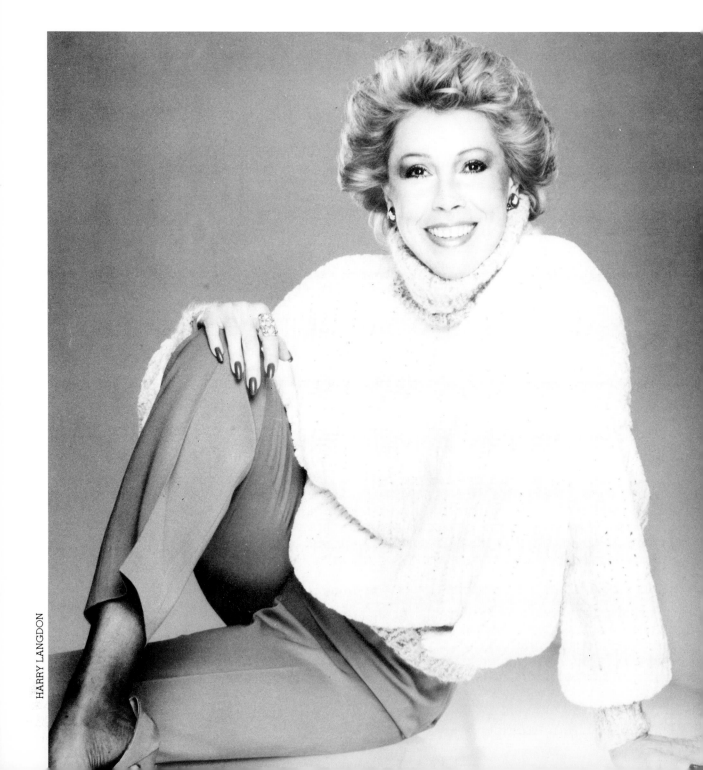

When you're in good physical condition, the heart—your human clock—works more efficiently. Your pulse rate is faster during exercise with a faster return to its normal resting rate. Blood rich in oxygen feeds your muscles and organs. The skin takes on a healthier glow. There is more spring in your step. These are the results of the program that appear long before there is a noticeable difference in the mirror. While other methods of exercise are fine, my method offers the chance for total improvement. This is what the Body Design by Gilda program will do for you.

Proper Muscle Tone, Increased Strength and Overall Firmness:

Muscle tone is one of the most important results of the program. Good muscle tone is achieved by increasing the amount of proteins in a muscle and an increase in the strength of the muscle fibers. This leads to more efficient body movements. Through training, the muscle will display a greater degree of tone, even in a resting state. The major part of the exercise portion of the Body Design by Gilda program involves muscle tension exercises isolating each muscle group and problem area with enough repetitions to cause additional strength and, therefore, more firmness. You will become a stronger and more active person.

Loss of Inches and a Decrease in Fat:

It is a proven fact that aerobic exercise tones muscles, defines muscles and alters their chemistry as well as increases the overall metabolic rate of the body.

Losing weight is not the issue, losing fat is the issue. One should strive to increase lean body mass. The lean body mass is the mass of the body minus the fat: only the muscle and bone. A lean body mass is what you want and the fat is what you strive to lose. Since muscle weighs more than fat, the overall body weight may not decrease as you begin to gain muscle and lose fat during exercise. The bathroom scale does not indicate improvement in lean body mass. The key to losing fat is to tip the calories burned/calories consumed balance so that we use more calories than we eat. Exercising burns calories but even more important, the aerobically fit body burns more calories at rest than the unfit body does.

The tape measure can be an inaccurate accounting of improved lean body mass as well. Take the thigh for instance. As you begin to exercise the thigh muscles, they tend to grow at first and the fat decreases. This can lead to no change in circumference. The space once occupied by the fat is now occupied by a bigger, more efficient muscle. As you continue to exercise the muscle itself loses its fat and becomes firm, and with proper stretching, it becomes shapely and slender.

Aerobic Improvement:

The aerobic principle of working the body at a pace that increases the oxygen intake and sustains the heart rate at 80 percent of its maximum level does strengthen heart, lungs and blood vessels. Even more important, aerobics improve the functioning of the muscles. The term cardiovascular conditioning has been replaced by aerobic conditioning because cardiovascular means heart and blood vessels. We now realize that endurance or aerobic-type exercises not only improve the heart and blood vessels, but to a greater extent make the muscles more efficient. In fact, the increases in muscular efficiency dwarf the improvements of the heart and blood vessels!

The well-conditioned muscle improves the quality of your life because the body is able to do more work without tiring. This type of exercise has been shown to result in a chemical secretion of endorphins throughout the body and the brain that results in an improved mental feeling and outlook. There seems to be a link to aerobic exercise and the endorphin release that results in an increase in self-esteem and a decrease in depression. Aerobics help you to move faster naturally. You will get more out of every day because you will be less tired.

More Flexibility and Suppleness:

The Body Design by Gilda program increases flexibility through a series of exercises that "gradually" stretch your muscles. It all starts with a careful warm-up that does just that—it warms up the body. An increased body temperature decreases the viscosity (thickness) of the fluids that lubricate the tissues and the joints. This helps to avoid injuries. The warm-up has the effect of loosening the tightness in the muscles, tissues and ligaments. This makes the beneficial stretching of these muscles, tissues and ligaments easier to achieve. All this improves posture, and makes the joints more supple. Every movement—from participating in sports activities to simply bending and tying your shoe—will be easier and more enjoyable. You will move gracefully. You will feel free and alive.

A Controlled Appetite:

Regular exercise can lead to a decrease, rather than an increase, in food consumption due to an exercise-inspired increase in the metabolic function. Latest medical findings indicate that even after a person has finished a planned exercise period, the metabolism (food and calorie-burning process) will not return to its normal level for several hours. This means that even when you are resting after exercise, the calories are still burning away. Regular exercise also alters your body chemistry so that your body is more apt to burn fats for energy and fewer calories convert into fat. In addition, immediately following physical exertion, blood sugar doesn't fluctuate as much, keeping those hunger pangs away for a longer period of time. You will be able to eat what you need without gaining fat.

Improved Relaxation:

The Body Design by Gilda program ends each exercise session with a planned period of mental and physical rest. This is extremely therapeutic and leaves you feeling refreshed and positive. So many of us have forgotten how good complete relaxation feels: the body has worked and earned the right to remain still and feel the new sensations pulsating through the developing muscles and stimulated tissues. This relaxation period is a first step toward learning to banish tension from every aspect of your daily life. It calms you emotionally.

And Always Energy Improves:

Many people are concerned that exercise will exhaust them and deplete their energy reserve. Just the opposite is true. Regular planned exercise actually gives you more energy. The Body Design by Gilda program helps you to break bad habits and replaces those habits with beneficial ones. As you start to energize and feel better, you become obsessed with improving still more.

Most of the time, a new student merely wants to get rid of some fat, but the program does a lot more than remove a few layers of unnecessary fat (and yes, there is *necessary* fat).

My program is a cycle of life. As you gain energy, you become more active. As you become more active, you burn more calories. As you become more active, you also exercise and tone the body. And exercise increases stamina and energy.

Many thousands of men and women have improved their health, their looks and their zest for living after making The Body Design by Gilda program their workout.

You can, too!

CHAPTER 3
THE SELF-APPRAISAL

The story is about you.

—HORACE

I have heard all the stories!

"I can't stand my thighs; I want them firmer . . . Every year I have to get a bigger belt size . . . How can I get my waistline back? . . . It has been a year since I had the baby and I still haven't gotten rid of my stomach . . . My rear end gets closer to the ground every year . . . I hate my arms and won't wear a sleeveless blouse."

Problems such as those start people exercising.

But those are very limited goals. Most people have the wrong mental attitude when they start to exercise seriously. They zero-in on a single area they want to improve. This means that they begin the program with the most limited viewpoint of what results to expect. After becoming involved with the Body Design by Gilda program, that same student soon forgets about that earlier limited goal. What the student wanted to fix in the first place gets fixed—along with everything else!

The student needs an attitude of unlimited potential when starting the program.

Jane Fonda had the right attitude. She had a great body when she first walked into my Beverly Hills studio back in 1978. She wanted to improve the overall tone of her body because she was filming a bikini sequence in the movie *California Suite.* Her stepmother, Shirlee Fonda, had been a student of mine and brought Jane to class one day. She soon understood the benefits of the program. She realized that it is a way of life and not just a temporary cure for a problem. The results are evident. She looks sensational and she has made the Body Design by Gilda her workout.

Reducing is only a part of what you should expect from the vigorous and stimulating effort that is required for an exercise program to be successful. You

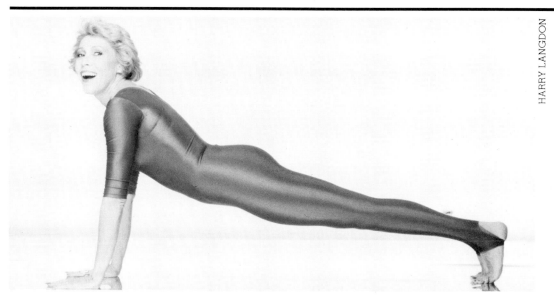

HARRY LANGDON

will work hard to lose those inches. You should be completely rewarded for all that effort. The Body Design by Gilda program is a challenge. But as the weeks pass you will find that you can accomplish more. Don't worry! Soon you will actually be looking forward to exercising every day.

So take a look at yourself and what you want for yourself.

Anyone who wants to look and feel great should make a realistic self-appraisal of the entire mental and physical condition before deciding what is needed from an exercise program. The benefits from a complete program are far more than the loss of inches and pounds. The Body Design by Gilda program is an exercise philosophy. The program is designed to become a part of every moment of your life. Besides improvement in physical appearance, the program offers the even more important potential for mental improvement. You will be nourishing your mind and body with the energy to thrive on the demands of your daily life.

When was the last time you jumped out of bed filled with energy? When was the last time you reached the end of the workday with lots of leftover energy? When was the last time you wanted to make love for hours?

Your high-energy time is coming.

Many people begin an exercise program with a poor attitude. They are positive that they will never look like Raquel Welch and will probably have four extra inches on those hips forever. They look at themselves in the mirror and see someone looking back who does not have promise. It all seems so hopeless.

But that is not what I see.

I watch men and women drag themselves into my class in the beginning. But after years of observing often spectacular improvement, I don't see them as fat, bloated and puffy. I look at their bone structure and mentally cut away the fat and sags and replace that drooping flesh with firm, toned muscle and smooth, taut skin. Most people would be surprised at just how much improvement they are capable of making.

Start a body appraisal by really looking at yourself in a full-length mirror. This is done without any clothes on. Yes, this unconcealed look at yourself can be painful, but it can also give you some hope.

Look at your height. Are you tall with long arms and legs, or short with short arms and legs, or somewhere in between? Often you will find that your wrists or ankles are still trim even though the legs and arms might have gathered some extra flesh.

Look at your body type. There are three different body types: endomorphic, mesomorphic and ectomorphic. *Endomorphic* bodies are characterized as round, soft, and smooth in contour with a predominance of abdomen, high, squared shoulders, and a short neck. *Mesomorphic* bodies have large bones covered with thick muscle with a comparatively slender waist. *Ectomorphics* are linear and fragile with small bones, thin muscles, and shoulders that tend to droop.

You should fit roughly into one of these categories. I say roughly, because most people are blends of body types. But every body type can be improved through a well-planned exercise program.

Look at your potentially worst areas. The buttocks! The arms! The thighs! The stomach! Imagine them firmer. Think how they will be in three months, six months, a year. Realize that the areas of the body you most want to improve will be the last to lose the fat. It is one of those sad facts of exercising life that fat seems to stay where you want it least. This is why some people are discouraged early in an exercise program when the weight seems to be coming off all the wrong places. The first weight lost is water. Padded areas have more fat to lose. You are probably losing weight evenly throughout the body, but those places with the extra padding have more pounds or inches to lose. Keep trying. You can lose it . . . where you want to lose it!

Mentally picture that body as you look at yourself in the mirror. Keep looking at yourself every day. I know this is hard when you have conditioned yourself to avoid looking at the body you have learned to ignore. Think more positively about that body as you improve. Think of your waist as slender. Think of your buttocks as well-rounded and hard. Think of your legs as sleek. Think of your neck as elegant. *Think of yourself as you want to be.*

Back to the reappraisal.

Hair can be attractive even on the most out-of-shape person. If your hair is poor, it can be improved after you have started exercising. This is because the stimulated blood flow (circulation) will improve the condition of the hair. I have seen hair so stimulated that it does thicken and occasionally reappear where it was thought to have been gone forever. Exercise stimulates the scalp oils that add shine to hair.

Exercise affects the entire body—including our eyes. During a workout, blood circulates at a greater rate throughout our bodies, opening the vessels in our eyes. When blood continually flows through those vessels, they remain open, thus reducing the opportunity for blockage to occur. A balance of good exercise, nutrition and sleep will promote healthy, strong eyes.

It is not so much the teeth that are affected by exercise but the gums. The oxygen-enriched blood that you are pumping through your body keeps the gums healthy.

Look at the face muscles. Is some of the bone structure still visible under the layer of extra fat that might be blurring the face? Imagine those cheekbones showing. Imagine a strong chinline. Imagine the puffiness gone from the face. Imagine that extra chin gone.

Stretch your neck and pull the chin in so that the head lies in a straight line perpendicular to the shoulders. Maybe you were permitting the neck (through poor posture) to drop forward and look shorter. This causes a double chin to form. Picture that neck as slender and graceful.

Pull your chest up high; allow your shoulders to relax and pull them into a squared, backward position (not hunched forward). You will probably notice an immediate improvement. Now think about how wonderful those straight and firm shoulders will be after you have strengthened the muscles that support the entire body.

A flabby upper arm can be tightened and reshaped into firm, sculptured and flexible muscle.

Hands might not seem capable of much change, but as you develop coordination while following the Body Design by Gilda program, hands do become more graceful and attractive. You feel and move more gracefully and this movement is reflected in the hands.

As the shoulders strengthen, the chest and pectoral muscles will reshape the contours of the chest and breasts. Improved posture will also help to make the chest areas of both men and women seem more attractive. While exercise does not usually make a woman's breasts increase, the improved posture and an increase of the mass of the pectoral muscles that support the breasts can make them more shapely and appear larger.

The back can be definitely improved both in appearance and health. As muscles strengthen and posture corrects, slumping disappears. Shoulders become squared instead of sagging. The back muscles can better support the stomach and chest muscles.

Those love handles at the waist will immediately begin to dwindle as your posture improves. If there are extra inches (sometimes the love handles are totally the result of poor posture), this fat will slowly disappear due to the exercise program and a good balanced diet.

The buttocks are one of the biggest problem areas. Because of biological and physiological differences, women tend to spread more than men. Women inherit additional protective fat here primarily for childbearing and have a tendency to develop problems if they don't keep this area exercised and toned. With the Body Design by Gilda program, it is possible to reshape the buttocks and lose those extra inches of fat. You probably have no idea what great buttocks are hiding behind you.

Most people neglect to work the stomach muscles. Unused stomach muscles give up. The result is a sagging belly that hangs over the belt or bulges through a dress. But there is hope. These muscles can be restrengthened (at any age), and those extra inches will disappear. As the muscle begins to tone and posture improves, the slack between the muscle and the skin starts to disappear. You will learn how to control the stomach muscles. You will learn how to exercise these muscles every moment of your life.

Those nasty fat cells seem to gather around the muscles of the outer and inner thighs. The Body Design by Gilda program emphasizes many variations of movements that help to convert the fat to muscle and to firm these seldom-used muscles. Seldom used, you say? Why, you walk all the time. Doesn't that do a lot for the thighs? Yes, walking does help the muscles on the front and back of the thighs and buttocks, but the limited movement of the leg while walking does little to tone the muscles on the sides of the upper leg. The program trains you to use these neglected muscles by developing an awareness of those important side motions and movements.

Some parts of the body are more difficult to improve than others. While arms might tone and firm quickly, the calves of the legs are usually a challenge. The calf does have potential, but acquiring fabulous calves means working hard. Muscles in the calf can be reshaped, however they tend to return to their original condition if not continually exercised. Calf improvement is a slow project, but certainly can be achieved.

The ankles are one of the most difficult areas of the body to change. The changes are usually subtle. Sometimes the ankle appears to be more shapely because of improvements of the calves and thighs. The line of the leg seems more graceful. (Maybe the ankles were always fine.) Yet, there is the possibility that the ankles are swollen because of poor posture, poor circulation, or being forced to carry around unnecessary weight.

Feet will be strengthened through exercising. Again, it is difficult to really alter the look of the foot, but proper posture and strengthening do make a difference to the condition of this all-so-important human foundation. Exercise will increase the strength of the arch and flexibility of the foot and toes.

Now you have done a head-to-toe reappraisal of yourself. I hope you are beginning to understand that every muscle in the body—our wonderful bodies—are interrelated. It is wrong to limit an improvement to a single goal like thin thighs or firmer buttocks. Firm, shapely buttocks start somewhere in the shoulder blades, and thin thighs have a definite relationship with strong stomach and back supporting muscles.

CHAPTER 4
COMMON SENSE AND NUTRITION

Diet: a way of living.

—WEBSTER

I do not believe in "miracle diets."

When it comes to dieting, there are no surefire, guaranteed miracles. Fad diets throw you into a temporary obsession with losing weight and are very unhealthy.

I want you to have a lifetime diet philosophy based on common sense and good nutrition. You cannot live on plantations of pineapple or oceans of chicken soup alone. The "quick weight loss" diets that promise "you will lose ten pounds in ten days" can be classified as fad diets. Every person loses weight at a different rate because each person's metabolism is unique.

Many fad diets temporarily adjust the metabolism, which causes a temporary loss of fluids and vital nutrients. Take a high-protein diet. The immediate weight loss a person experiences from this diet is water loss. High-protein diets throw the body's metabolism out of balance and can cause unneeded stress and tension, often causing calcium depletion, dehydration, nausea and fatigue. The average female needs approximately 44 grams of protein a day, depending on her size and weight. Any protein beyond the body's daily requirement is stored as fat. Too much protein and not enough other nutrients in the diet can deplete the carbohydrates stored in the muscles. The dieter will then experience a lack of energy.

A sensibly balanced diet does not upset the metabolism; it actually helps it to function more efficiently. Your metabolism is the inner chemistry of your body, which changes the digested nutrients (foods) you have consumed into energy to meet the body's requirements. Exercise can regulate your metabolism and make it more efficient. In addition to burning calories during a workout, your body continues to consume calories at a higher rate for up to six hours after exercising. The best exercise to produce an increase in metabolic efficiency is aerobics.

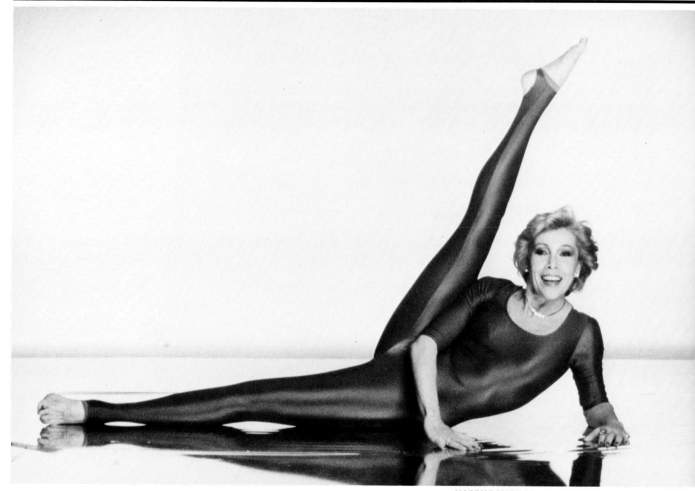

HARRY LANGDON

The basis of the Body Design by Gilda philosophy is: *The Calories You Take into Your Body Will Become Extra Weight and Be Stored as Fat if They Are Not Used up Through Activity.* The Body Design by Gilda program will help you metabolize approximately 300 to 500 calories per hour, depending on your body size and weight.

Through exercise you can decrease the amount of fat stored throughout every part of the body. This includes not only the visible fat in the stomach, thighs and upper arms, but even more important, that invisible fat that hides in the muscles. A newborn calf is mostly muscle, but a beef-producing adult animal that has been kept on a feedlot will develop a high concentration of fat in its muscles. This produces the marbling that is so highly praised in quality beef. Unfortunately, the same thing happens to people.

Besides proper exercise, the body needs proper nourishment.

You need to start listening to your body's needs. This "instinctive" understanding of your urges and cravings will make you more aware of what will become your individual diet philosophy.

I don't believe there will ever be a "perfect diet" that is right for everyone. I do believe that you have to develop a realistic eating pattern to maintain good health. *Learn to Become Aware of the Needs of Your Body!*

. . . and what are those important needs?

The necessary nutrients consist of: proteins, fats, carbohydrates, vitamins, minerals and water.

Protein Nutrients: These are found in meats, fish, poultry, eggs, dairy products and some whole grains. A healthy eating pattern should include a daily intake of ten to 15 percent protein. Most people consume far more protein in their diets than their bodies require . . . and the unused protein will be converted into fat.

Fat Nutrients: Found in meats, meat skins, oils, butter, cheeses and cookies or cakes. About 30 percent of your daily calorie intake should be fats. It is estimated that the average American diet is 40 to 45 percent fat. Fats provide the fuel to energize the body; however, unused fat is stored in the body just as that—fat. The good news is that this stored fat can be transformed into energy through exercising.

Carbohydrate Nutrients: Found in fruits, grains, cereals and vegetables. Carbohydrates, your main source of energy, should provide about 60 percent of your daily calorie intake. The principal carbohydrates present in most foods are sugars, starches and cellulose. There are two kinds of sugars: simple sugars (found in honey and fruits), which are easy to digest, and refined sugars (table sugar), which are more difficult to digest.

Starches (also known as complex carbohydrates) are found in whole grains, breads and crackers. These starches, besides providing energy, provide us with fiber. Fiber is not digested by the human body. It plays a very important role in keeping our elimination system working properly. Foods high in fiber, such as complex carbohydrates, are also an excellent source of vitamins and minerals.

Cellulose is the nondigestible fiber found in the skins of fruits, vegetables and whole grains. It is a very valuable component of the human diet. Cellulose causes the body to absorb more water, thus making elimination easier.

Refined sugars (carbonated drinks, candy, cakes, pies, etcetera) are absorbed into the bloodstream very fast and provide "quick" energy. This is not energy that lasts. Have you ever eaten a candy bar and shortly thereafter felt tired? This is because you've experienced a fast drop in your blood sugar, and you actually have less energy than before you ate it! Complex carbohydrates (breads, crackers and cereals) are absorbed much slower, providing you with a sustained energy level throughout the day.

I advise that you add extra complex carbohydrates to your diet to maintain your energy level, if you participate in a regular exercise program.

Vitamins and Minerals: There is a lot of confusion about vitamins and minerals. For the most part, a well-balanced diet should provide all the vitamins and minerals that are necessary. Taking huge doses of vitamins is a waste. The body absorbs only what it requires and disposes of the rest. Since most of us do not make the effort to eat a well-balanced diet, a vitamin and mineral supplement might be necessary.

Water: I always try to drink a minimum of eight to ten glasses of water a day. I keep a thermos bottle filled with pure water on my desk. By keeping that thermos nearby, I make sure that I always get the needed liquid in my system. *Do not* count other liquids such as coffee, tea, juice, milk or soda pop as part of your pure water intake. Those liquids contain other elements that do not cleanse the body like clear water.

Water makes up approximately two-thirds of our body's weight and plays a major role in our overall health. It's essential for carrying waste materials out of the body . . . it's responsible for maintaining a normal body temperature, cooling us down by perspiring . . . and it is water that maintains the tissue balance of our skin. It is easy to see that we could not survive without water!

Your environment and the amount of your physical activity dictates what your rate of water loss will be. Each individual varies, depending on where they live and what they do during each day. *Example:* If you live in Phoenix, Arizona, and play tennis every day, your water loss will be greater than someone who lives in Anchorage, Alaska, and spends most of the day inside. The average adult loses approximately three quarts of water daily through excretion and perspiration.

I'd like to share the eating program that has worked for me. The program contains a wide enough variety of foods to choose from to maintain a healthy menu and satisfy your individual preferences.

GILDA'S REGIME

BREAKFAST SELECTIONS	I choose one from each group. You may mix and match any protein with any carbohydrate group.

Fruit Group: *(carbohydrates)*	6 ounces of fresh-squeezed orange juice, 75 calories
	or
	1 piece of fresh fruit, 60–80 calories

Grain Group: *(carbohydrates)*	1 cup of oatmeal with 2 tablespoons of raisins, 227 calories
	or
	whole-grain toast, 60–90 calories per slice
	or
	½ bran muffin or ½ bagel, 60–80 calories
	or
	1 ounce heated tortilla, 110 calories
	or
	1 cup cold cereal, 110 calories

Protein Group:	1 egg (scrambled without butter, poached or hard-boiled), 80 calories
	or
	½ cup cottage cheese, 120 calories
	or
	8 ounces of plain low-fat yogurt, 150 calories
	or
	½ cup of low-fat milk, 60 calories

(*Note:* All calorie counts are approximations)

LUNCH SELECTIONS

Grain Group:
1 slice of whole-grain bread, 60–90 calories

or

a bagel, 165 calories

Protein Group:
4 ounces white-meat turkey, 200 calories
4 ounces white-meat chicken, 200 calories
4 ounces water-packed tuna, 150 calories
1 egg, 80 calories
¼ of an avocado, 95 calories
1 ounce hard cheese, 100 calories

or

a "light hand" peanut butter and jelly sandwich. But, remember, *no* spoonfuls before. 50 calories per tablespoon for the jelly; 90 calories per table-spoon for the peanut butter.

Fruits and Vegetables:
a fruit salad, approximately 80 calories per cup

or

a bean salad, 270 calories per cup

or

a vegetable salad with any of the following:
lettuce, 10 calories per cup
celery stalk, 7 calories
½ cup sliced green peppers, 9 calories
radishes, 7 calories for four small radishes
spinach, 9 calories per cup
carrots, 21 calories per carrot
onions, 4 ounces, 4 calories

or

any of the green leafy vegetables low in calories

DINNER SELECTIONS

Carbohydrate Group:	½ of a baked potato, 50 calories *or* ⅔ cup rice, 133 calories *or* 1 cup pasta, 200 calories
Vegetables:	either a small green salad *or* 1 cup of cooked (steamed) vegetables, approximately 40–50 calories
Protein Group:	4 ounces salmon (in water), 160 calories 4 ounces shrimp, scallops, 120 calories 4 ounces halibut or swordfish, 200 calories *or* beef, 4 ounces, 250 calories (ground brisket, steak or roast, lean only) *or* 6 ounces white-meat chicken, 300 calories 6 ounces white-meat turkey, 300 calories (always eat chicken, Cornish hens and turkey without the skin)
Fat Group:	1 tablespoon of butter (100 calories) on potato or to sauté fish *or* 1 tablespoon mayonnaise, 105 calories *or* 1 tablespoon safflower oil, 128 calories
DESSERT SELECTIONS	1 baked apple with honey and cinnamon, 95 calories *or* 4 ounces frozen yogurt, 150 calories *or* 1 slice angel food cake, 70 calories

SNACKS CONSIST OF ANY OF THE FOLLOWING:

2 cups mixed vegetables, 75 calories

or

1 hard-boiled egg, 80 calories

or

2 ounces lean chicken or turkey or 1 ounce of cheese, 100 calories

or

4 to 5 crackers, 95 calories

or

1 slice of bread, 60–90 calories

or

1 piece of fruit or 6 ounces of fruit juice, 60–80 calories

or

½ bagel, 85 calories

or

½ muffin, 60 calories

or

1 ounce raisins, 85–90 calories

or

melba toast with 2 teaspoons of peanut butter, 75 calories

or

½ cup of low-fat milk, 60 calories

or

1 ounce of plain popcorn, 109 calories

or

8 to 10 nuts (almonds, cashews, peanuts, pecans), 70 calories

In the two decades I've spent working with people, I've never met anyone that didn't have some favorite indulgences—and that includes food, drink and sex!

I'm not going to tell you never to eat a piece of chocolate-fudge cake, when that piece of cake really gives you pleasure and satisfaction. You should realize that piece of cake contains approximately 500 calories. You must burn up those calories during the day by adding activity or by cutting calories somewhere else. With this balance, you will transform that piece of chocolate-fudge cake from what could negatively be a weight gain, to something positive. By adding, for instance, an aerobic exercise class, you have enjoyed your splurge, and your body has the benefit of an extra dose of constructive exercise.

One of my students, Sandra Theodore, is an example of a beautiful woman who really loves to eat. She is one of the most popular *Playboy* centerfolds. Besides being high-energy, life around the *Playboy* mansion also can be highly caloric, so Sandra maintains a rigorous exercise program that balances her sometimes high-calorie diet with calorie-burning exercises.

Here are some of my favorite indulgences. These goodies are not only listed with their calories, but also with the amount of activity necessary to use up those calories. (This is based on the weight of a 125-pound woman. These figures are approximate, as your calorie expenditure can vary greatly depending on your individual body structure and weight. The more you weigh, the more calories you burn during the same exercise period.)

1 quarter-pound hamburger with bun (454 calories)—Roller-skate for 1 hour and 35 minutes.

1 hot dog with bun (354 calories)—Vigorously square dance for 1 hour.

half of a 10-inch pizza pie (436 calories)—Scrub floors for 1 hour and 15 minutes.

1 ounce of potato chips (160 calories)—Golf for 35 minutes.

10 french fries (150 calories)—Dance vigorously for 30 minutes. (For a full order of fries, enter a marathon dance contest!)

1 small avocado (390 calories)—Go bicycling for 1 hour.

1 tablespoon Thousand Island dressing (100 calories)—Water-ski for 15 minutes.

1 12-ounce can of beer (155 calories)—Do housework for 50 minutes.

Martini cocktail (160 calories)—Wash windows for 50 minutes.

4 chocolate chip cookies (212 calories)—Nonstop gardening for 1 hour.

1 glazed doughnut (150 calories)—Go bowling for 30 minutes.

3-inch wedge of coconut cake (400 calories)—Play vigorous tennis for 50 minutes.

1 chocolate bar (300 calories)—Making love for 15 minutes burns off approximately 60 calories (depending on intensity of the lover, of course!!). You'd have to make love for 1½ hours to burn off that chocolate bar!! My suggestion is to get a strong lover, with a lot of stamina and in great physical condition!! It might be worth it!

I will never forget the evening I went to a very exclusive restaurant in Beverly Hills. One of my students was having dinner—she was "indulging" in fettuccine Alfredo. The minute she saw me, she dumped the entire meal on the floor! I told her it would have been easier if she'd just come to class the next day!

There's no way of getting around the fact that if you love to eat, you must balance those calories with activity. Otherwise, you're going to gain weight. The more activity you put into your life, the more you can eat the wonderful foods you enjoy! Most people aren't aware of the fact that simple, everyday activities like driving to work, taking an elevator or walking down the hall, burn calories.

The more activity you incorporate into your day, the more calories you will burn! Here are a few examples. (Again based on an average 125-pound woman.)

Active Person	Calories Expended	Sedentary Person	Calories Expended
Does morning stretches, 10 minutes	25	Drives to work; total time 13 minutes	32
Walks to work (briskly), carrying briefcase; 1.5 miles in 23 minutes	100	Takes elevator to office	7
Walks up two flights of stairs to office	35	Eats lunch in company room down the hall	36
Walks to and from lunch, ¼ mile each way (2 m.p.h.)	45	Drives home from work	32
Walks home from work; 1.5 miles in 23 minutes	100	Drives through fast-food restaurant for dinner	13
Body Design by Gilda Exercise Program	390*		
Grocery shopping, lifting bags into and out of car, total time 1 hour	210		
1 hour of basic housecleaning	210		
	1,115		120

Total *Extra* Calories
Utilized by Adding
Activities to Your Day

*Expenditure will vary depending on how vigorous the workout.

Common Sense

1. Eat three meals a day and two to three "light" snacks to keep your blood sugar up.

2. Food and your emotional relationship to food should be put into the proper perspective. *Don't live to eat . . . but eat to live—healthy!*

3. Eat slowly and eat the right combinations of food groups.

4. Always dine in an eating area. Never snack in bed or in front of the television where outside influences can distract you from being aware of the amount of food you are consuming.

5. Don't eat when you're not hungry . . . and don't wait until you're starving or you will overeat.

6. Drink eight to ten glasses of pure water a day (and don't count other beverages, such as coffee, tea, juices, milk, diet drinks, etcetera).

7. Do eat fresh fruits, such as apples, bananas (my favorite), oranges, grapes, nectarines, plums, mangoes, melons, pears, pineapples, grapefruits, peaches, papayas, apricots, strawberries, blueberries, raspberries, kiwi, cherries, tangerines and prunes. Always eat three to four servings of fruit a day. (A serving is not necessarily the *whole* fruit) i.e., half of a banana is considered a whole fruit serving.

8. Eat several high-vitamin cooked and raw vegetables, such as lima beans, beets, split peas, pinto beans, garbanzo beans, lentils, kidney beans . . . also, broccoli, asparagus, carrots, cauliflower, celery, chard, cucumbers, eggplant, mushrooms, okra, onions, parsley, radishes, lettuce, sprouts, spinach, leeks, turnips, jicama, tomatoes, green peppers, scallions, squash, peas, cabbage, brussels sprouts, dandelions, kale, endive, watercress, rutabaga, pea pods and artichokes.

Helpful Hints

1. Try to eat pure foods, without heavy seasonings and sauces. Don't camouflage the true taste of foods.

2. Satisfy your cravings and urges, they're realistic!! Just don't binge, only eat half of what you are craving instead of the whole thing.

3. Save up some extra calories during the day when you know that you will be going out to dinner that night.

4. Have a little snack *before* you go to a cocktail party.

5. *Don't* let your blood sugar drop.

6. If you desire an alcoholic drink, first drink a whole glass of pure or mineral water; then have your cocktail. A white wine spritzer is best; half wine and half soda water—it's really refreshing!

7. Don't use extra salt. There is ample salt in today's foods to fulfill anyone's salt requirements.

8. Eat less meat high in fats, such as beef, pork, veal and lamb.

9. Do eat more fish instead of fat-laden animal meats.

10. Eat more turkey and chicken, but, take the skin off first.

11. Bake, broil, steam or poach foods; avoid fats and oils.

12. Try to avoid all fried foods. No fried chicken and french fries.

13. Use low-fat or non-fat dairy products. I love to use yogurt as a salad dressing base or as a dip for raw vegetables.

14. Avoid fast-food hamburgers, hot dogs, breaded fried fish, and cold cuts such as salami, pastrami and corned beef.

15. Start to develop a taste for lemon and vinegar as a salad dressing.

16. Keep an eye on the size of your food portions. Try to cook smaller amounts of foods. Fill each plate in the kitchen instead of covering the dining table with enticing serving dishes heaped with food.

17. Discipline yourself so that you become calorie aware and try to stay within your calorie goal.

18. Remember beverages, especially alcoholic, have calories too.

19. Cancel your membership to The Clean Plate Club!!!

You Must Become Constantly Vigilant of What Your Eating Patterns Are Doing to You.

There is no perfect diet philosophy for everyone. You must create your own philosophy. You must learn to understand your own body's needs. As you become more familiar with your own muscles and your own energy levels, you will realize what diet philosophy is right for your body. Give your body the chance to function properly. Then you will have your own philosophy for success.

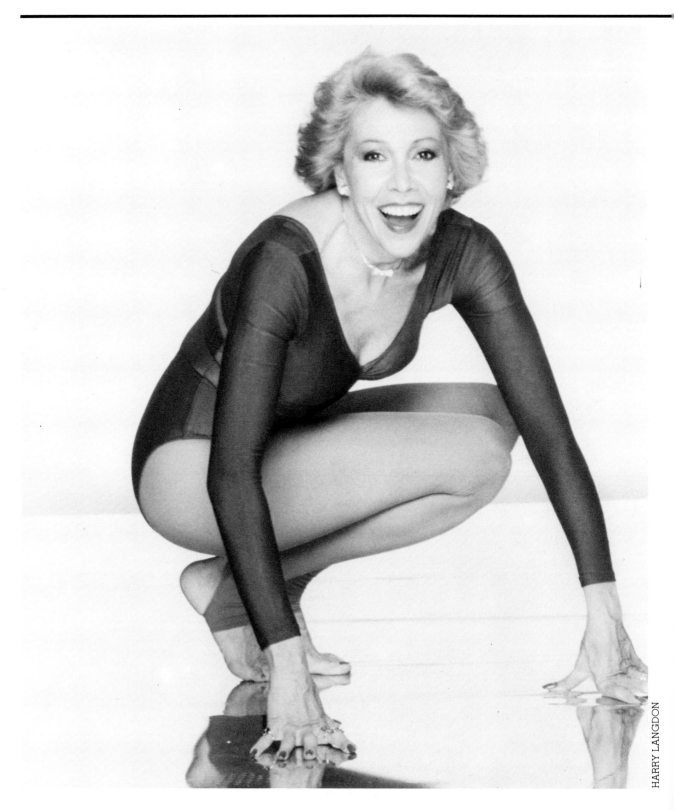

HARRY LANGDON

CHAPTER 5
WAKE UP TURNED-ON

Let us be up and doing.

—LONGFELLOW

You must have quality rest!

If you are going to commit to an exercise program as a way of life, you will have to fuel that program with proper rest. Proper rest gives you the energy to exercise. The way you feel the first few minutes after awakening has a lot to do with how you will function for the rest of the day. If you wake up tired, if you have to drag yourself from the warmth and security of the bed, or if you try to avoid waking up at all, you need to learn how to sleep and wake up properly.

Sleep and exercise are dependent upon each other. Sleep prepares the body for exercise. Exercise prepares the body for sleep. This is a cycle. Proper sleep is the basic ingredient of the I-am-ready-to-leap-out-of-bed-and-greet-the-day morning ritual. Few of us put much effort into planning and orchestrating proper sleep. We think that getting under the blankets and closing the eyes and waiting for sleep is enough. That is not enough.

The body must be primed and ready for really beneficial sleep. I follow a sleep ritual that couples the benefits of sleep-inducing physical activity with the proper resting procedure. This program not only produces a sound sleep that rests the muscles but a satisfying sleep that eases the tensions of the mind.

The program starts the night before.

It is most important to be mentally and physically relaxed when going to bed. There should be no tensions from the strains of the previous day. There should be no lingering memories of problems and worries. Sometimes a luxurious hot bath or some soothing music is enough to relax the mind that is racing with the thoughts of a demanding day. Many people relax by sitting in front of the faint glow of the television set while their minds drift and their bodies sink deep into a comfortable chair. All these things can promote relaxation. But you must make an effort to relax *before* getting into bed. The winding down period must be accomplished away from the sheets. The bed should be reserved for sleeping, not worrying.

You know the feeling.

You get into bed aching for rest. Suddenly the eyes are wide open. The mind is racing. Instead of a resting place, the bed becomes a brooding area where all the difficulties and frustrations of the day are re-examined.

Before going to bed, relax your body with some soothing exercises. Do some gentle stretching. Avoid strenuous movements such as calisthenics and aerobics. Demanding exercises only stimulate the heart rate and excite the mind and body. *A Gilda Rule: Never Do Vigorous Exercising Before Going to Sleep.*

The exercises in the Back Release section of this book are perfect for removing the tensions from the back and neck. Since I love to walk, I recommend a short stroll (at a slow pace instead of a gallop) in the night air. Enjoy the quiet. Soon you will be ready to go to bed.

Here are some considerations to follow that will help you to fall asleep faster, sleep better, and awaken refreshed and eager to meet the demands of a new day.

- The mattress is crucial to great sleep. When buying a mattress, you have to test it. Yes, this means going to a store and climbing into bed. Note whether the mattress pushes firmly but with resilience against the hips and shoulders. A mattress that is too soft or too hard (yes, extra-extra firm is not always extra-extra good) forces muscles to work constantly to straighten the spine. Sit on the edge of the bed. Sturdy mattress edges are a sign of quality. And remember to turn your mattress periodically to preserve its support.

- Sleep in a quiet place. Even though you might not be awakened by outside noises, you are aware of them. Sounds act as subliminal stimuli that keep us from staying in a deep sleep. The effect of noise far outlasts the length of the noise period. Many sleep studies have proved that even if a person is not awakened by outside noises, the quality of the sleep is damaged. And the sleeper who was subconsciously disturbed functions less efficiently the following day.

- Temperature affects sleep. Most people think they sleep better in a slightly cooler environment of about 65 degrees Fahrenheit. One study showed that people do awaken more often when temperatures were above 75 degrees. But one study also showed that dreams became more emotional and unpleasant as temperatures dropped below the middle 60s.

- Keep lots of fresh air circulating in the room. Fresh oxygen-rich air is very important to sleeping.

- Posture is important even while sleeping. Orthopedic experts recommend that if you sleep on your back, it is wise to keep the legs slightly bent. You might try putting a pillow under the knees. This will help to relax the back. Everyone can remember awakening from a sound sleep because of the stabbing pain of a cramp. A properly placed pillow can help to ease the strain on muscles that might otherwise experience this problem. An excellent sleeping position is to lie on your side with the hips and knees slightly bent and the body weight concentrated on the pelvis. Avoid high piles of pillows; this places strain on the neck, arms and shoulders. Avoid sleeping flat on your back if you have any history of back problems.

- Who you sleep with makes a difference. Notice, I use the term "sleep." Who you stay awake with in bed is another consideration. But say there are two of you in bed and you are both attempting to sleep; select your partner carefully. Recent studies have shown that sleep is a communicative process. Couples mirror the actions of each other. If one moves, the other will soon after. Very affectionate people tend to gravitate toward each other and snuggle. When a person is very physical, that person will be very physical during sleep. This is fine if both partners are equally affectionate or physical. Alas, this is seldom the case. So often, one partner will make a move into the other partner's personal space, and the other partner will roll away. All this chasing and rolling can cause sleep to lose quality. Sometimes the answer is twin beds.

- Think pleasant thoughts before going to sleep. Think about the nice things that happened during the day. If nothing nice happened during the day, think about anything you have ever enjoyed. Think about what you would like to accomplish in the future. Think pleasant.

- Don't binge on alcohol and food before going to bed. It is difficult to rest when the stomach is singing *The Star-Spangled Banner* and your tongue is saluting the flag. Avoid protein-laden foods before sleeping because these are fuel foods that rev-up the body. Gas and bloat-causing foods such as carbonated beverages and certain fruits such as cantaloupes can interrupt the sleep pattern. Even that nighttime tradition, a glass of milk, can produce chemical reactions that disturb sleep. While it is a good idea to have some food in the stomach to give those stomach acids something to do during the night, keep that food something simple such as Jell-O, toast and herb tea. Try to wake up hungry for breakfast instead of feeling filled from the night before.

Here is how I sleep:

First, I let myself sense the soothing warmth of the bed. Make the bed a comforting and pleasant place to be at the end of the day.

Second, I let my legs move apart (keeping knees slightly bent) and concentrate on releasing all the tension in my legs and feet.

Third, I let this sense of relaxation seep through the rest of my body.

Fourth, I keep thinking only pleasant thoughts until sleep comes. Never clutter your sleep with the difficult memories of the day. Find something cheerful and hopeful to occupy your mind.

When morning arrives and the alarm rings (my sleep schedule is so well planned that I usually awaken naturally and seldom need to set an alarm), I reverse the process to start the blood circulating. I do not immediately jump out of bed. It is nice to wake up slowly.

The first thing I think about when my eyes open in the morning is the feet. I stretch the legs and start circling the feet toward each other to loosen the joints in the ankles. Then I reverse the direction of the circle. About ten circles in each direction will be enough to stimulate the blood flow in the extremities of the feet.

Then I flex the ankles while pointing the toes toward my nose and then toward the foot of the bed. Ten of these flexes should start the blood circulating.

The feet are now awake.

The knees are next. While still laying on the back, bend both knees. This will lift the covers off the bed. Then straighten the legs. This stretches the front of the thighs. Repeat this movement about four times.

Next, roll over onto the right side and bring the knees to the chest. This helps to stretch the entire back and neck and release any tension that might be in the lower spine. Do several of these exercises on each side. This can help to relax a tight back, especially if there has been any tension or stress during the night such as a nightmare or restlessness due to worry.

Now take the covers off.

Roll both legs over to the side of the bed and place both feet on the floor. Take a few deep breaths. Lean forward with the head and shoulders positioned facing the floor. Straighten the body up. Open your eyes wide. Squeeze them shut tightly. Keep repeating this until the eyes feel very clear and bright.

Move the legs approximately two feet apart, lean forward, and place the hands palms down on the floor. The blood will flow toward the head.

This is the first moment of exercise for the muscles in the back of the leg. Do everything slowly. Stretch the hamstring muscles and buttocks. No need to rush and possibly strain something.

Always be alert to feel the muscles stretching and exerting but do not push to the point of pain. There is a vast difference between the benefit a muscle receives from stretching and the results of pushing a muscle beyond its early-morning tolerance level.

If you require more stimulation to start your day, here are another five minutes' worth of wake-up exercises. I realize that many people will want to do only the bare minimum morning wake-up exercises, so I don't force the issue with too many exercises before the shower and coffee (better yet, herb tea).

But just in case!

To loosen the neck and shoulders, lie on your back with legs extended and straight (not stiff). The body should be relaxed and comfortable. Place hands behind the head with the elbows off to the side. Then bring the elbows together, lift the head, and gently roll the chin forward to the chest. Then relax back to the first position. Repeat a few times.

To begin warming up the lower back and hips, lie on your back, extend the right leg and bend the left knee toward your chest. Hold for eight counts. Release slowly while extending the left leg and bending the right knee for another eight counts.

The way you get out of bed is also important. Don't bolt out of bed. Ease your sleepy back and body away from the comfort of the warm mattress and blankets. Lie on your back with arms and legs both straight in a natural position. While bending your knees slightly, slowly roll onto one side of the bed. One arm will be underneath you. With the other arm, place the palm of the hand (palm down) on the bed in front of your chest. Using that hand and arm as a lever, push yourself up first on the elbows and then with both arms supporting your weight. You should now be in a sitting position. Place both feet on the floor and sit on the edge of the mattress with the back straight. Slowly roll the chin to the chest, then vertebra by vertebra continue curling the head to the knees.

Then reverse the process to the upright position, keeping the chin tucked until the spine is uncurled.

Now get up.

A lot of you are probably saying: "I don't have time for all that exercise stuff."

You do have time. Think about those minutes after the alarm goes off when you usually try to linger awhile under the covers half awake and half asleep. Fill those minutes with life-giving morning movement. Get yourself going on the right track. Give yourself a good start. It's going to be a great day!

CHAPTER 6
THE IMPROVEMENT ATMOSPHERE

He who has begun has half done.

Dare to be wise; begin.

—HORACE

Let nothing get in the way of your success!

The commitment to an exercise program begins long before you do that first leg lunge or sit-up. The commitment begins when you decide to create an exercise atmosphere in your life. The correct exercise atmosphere not only helps you to get the most benefit from your effort, but makes you actually want to exercise.

This will require some reorganization of your life. Certainly having the proper clothing, the correct equipment and a planned schedule for exercising is important. But maintaining an I-am-not-going-to-let-anything-get-in-the-way-of-my-success attitude is even more important.

Life is filled with interruptions. From the moment you awake, there will always be something or someone ready to stick a foot in front of you in an effort to trip up your exercise ambitions. You have to make the time in your life for an exercise schedule. I know this is difficult. We are all chasing the clock. We are all overwhelmed by the demands for our time. This is something that you must give to yourself . . . a piece of time to make your life have more quality.

You can find that time. Think of all those precious wasted minutes in your day: that unnecessary phone call; those coffee and cigarette breaks; that pointless little argument with a family member or co-worker. Add all those wasted minutes together and you will find time to exercise.

- Use your lunch break as an exercise break. A light lunch of fruit, salad or juice will be worked off by the exercising.
- Instead of fighting rush hour traffic, try to find a convenient place to exercise and start your journey home a little later. This helps to eliminate stress.

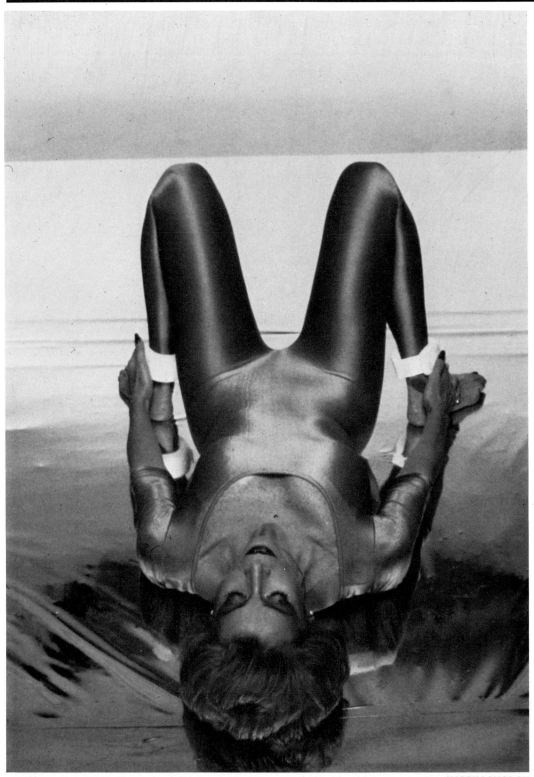

HARRY LANGDON

- If you have children, find a friend and take turns watching the children. This will free time for exercising in both households.
- Get the children to exercise with you during your quality family time.
- Decide to stop watching certain television shows and fill that time with exercising. Or exercise while you are watching TV.

See, you *can* find the time for exercising.

Many people, including myself, prefer to exercise in the morning. This exercise session immediately gives me a shot of energy that I need to take me through the day. It gets the oxygen flowing through my bloodstream to my muscles. It turns me on. I begin to generate energy.

But if you are not a morning person or your work schedule interferes, arrange the exercise times whenever you want. Just be sure that you do the Body Design by Gilda program on a regular basis, a minimum of one hour every other day. It would be best to do the program every day, but if that is impossible, try to do at least 20 to 30 minutes of stretching and aerobics daily.

Eat lightly before exercising. Allow at least one hour for the blood to assist the stomach in digesting before you call upon it to oxygenate your muscles during exercise.

Create the proper atmosphere for exercising.

Be sure that you have cleared enough body movement space so that legs and arms will not be bumping into furniture. Stand and extend the arms in every direction. Then lie down and extend both the arms and legs. Usually an area about seven feet square is ample space.

The area you select for working out should be well ventilated. *A Gilda Rule: Don't Ever Work Out in a Closed Room.* You need lots of fresh oxygen from that circulating air. Working outside is wonderful. I strongly disagree with other exercise programs that recommend exercising in a hot and closed room. You do not want to overheat your body. Overperspiring can cause dizziness and heat exhaustion and deplete the body of its energy. Circulating fresh air helps to prevent overheating.

Play upbeat tempo music to excite and stimulate your body movements. This makes exercising more fun. You feel inspired like a dancer. Since my exercise program is designed to be performed like a dance routine, music is an absolute must. Keep changing the music. Maybe some rock today. A Charleston tomorrow.

If it is possible to have the luxury of working in front of a mirror, the ability to watch yourself is most beneficial to exercising. The mirror can be your partner and teacher. It can show you whether you are positioning the body correctly. It will always be there reflecting your improvements. Make the person in the mirror your teacher:

—Let the person in the mirror help you to stretch.
—Let the person in the mirror inspire you.
—Let the person in the mirror be your exercise companion.
—Let the person in the mirror make you confident.

Sylvester Stallone and Susan Anton proved my point. My penthouse studio in Beverly Hills is mirrored on one wall and windowed on two walls overlooking a magnificent view of all of Los Angeles. They wanted private Body Design lessons. They watched each other while exercising. But finally, they started looking at themselves in the mirror. Your best exercise partner is yourself even if you are with someone as handsome as Sly Stallone or as beautiful as Susan Anton.

You need a matlike padded surface on the floor to provide the back with proper cushioning. A towel should be placed over the mat to absorb perspiration.

A banister, a countertop or a sturdy chair can serve as a barre for the ballet portion of the Body Design by Gilda program. The barre should be no higher than the height of your hips. The idea in barre movements is to allow the muscle to stretch and relax in a non-weightbearing, unstrained position. Too high a barre will not permit the muscle to properly relax. If the muscle cannot properly relax, it can't elongate. The chair, banister or counter must be very sturdy so that it will not tip over.

As you progress in the arm and leg sections of the program, you might buy some light ankle weights to add additional resistance (one-to-five-pound tops). Ankle weights with Velcro closures can be used on the wrists. Caution: Do not use weights if you have any history of back or knee problems.

That is all the physical equipment that is needed.

How you look is important. From the beginning of an exercise program, women want to look as attractive as possible. (Yes, I said "women" because most men are perfectly happy in their shorts, T-shirts and sweat pants.)

Don't be afraid to wear a leotard. So many women are hesitant to put their bodies into leotards and tights because they feel these close-fitting garments are too revealing. Actually, a properly designed leotard should be supportive, should be contoured to fit properly, and can be very flattering.

This reminds me of Bette Midler.

One day I looked at the back of my class and saw Bette Midler with arms, legs and everything flying. She was having a wonderful time. She was also wearing one of the leotards I had designed.

After the class a panting Divine Miss M bounced up to me and said, "I absolutely adored this workout and this leotard is great. It is the first leotard that was ever able to support my chest." To a leotard designer, that was the ultimate challenge and the ultimate compliment.

I was a dancer. I know there is a reason why these garments have always been an important part of the dancer's life; they fit and follow the grace and balance of the dancer's body. Properly designed leotards and tights will contour, support and conceal figure faults such as a wide waist, heavy thighs, full hips and veined legs.

Flexatard support tights are particularly flattering to a woman's legs. By the time most women are in their mid-twenties, small veins can begin to appear beneath the skin. The support tights hide these veins while shaping the leg muscles. They give the leg a firm appearance.

It is important to buy a high-quality leotard and tights. Tug at the seams to see if they are tightly sewn. Try on the leotard and move around while watching whether the fabric tends to stretch over the body. You are purchasing a leotard for action and it should be up to the demands of a vigorous exercise program.

Leotards have a tendency to shrink. The 100-percent cotton leotards can shrink the most. The cotton-polyester blends shrink less. The 100-percent nylon leotards are loose fitting and lack support. But nylon and spandex blends are supportive and wear best. Blends of cotton and spandex also support and wear well, and the blends of cotton, polyester and spandex are the best of the cotton blends. You will need to experiment to find which fabric is right for your body.

Always follow the washing instructions that come with your leotard and tights. If you understand how to take care of your leotards and tights they will last for years. Always wash them in the mildest soaps and wash them by themselves. Immediately after wearing a leotard, soak it in tepid water, or at least rinse out the high perspiration areas. Then rinse it in cold water. Get out all the soaps and chemicals. If you use a dryer, use the light cycle. I prefer that leotards be drip-dried. This helps them to retain their original shape. Most people just throw their leotards and tights into the wash with the towels and other laundry and dry them in the hot cycle. This can shrink the elastic in the garments as much as 50 percent. Having a leotard suddenly be a size smaller can come as an unpleasant shock to the person who has been watching her diet and carefully exercising to lose unwanted inches.

While exercise and health have always been the most important part of my career, I noticed while looking at my exercise classes, that there were no fashionable and attractive-looking leotards. This gave me the idea to start designing leotards that supported, flattered and fit the body properly. So in 1975, I began designing the Flexatard leotard. I wanted to create a beautiful garment that would inspire my students to want to exercise. The Flexatard was my idea of a uniform for exercise success. Today Flexatard, Inc., is a multi-million-dollar company.

Women want to have style while exercising. They want colors. Don't be afraid of wearing colors even though your body might not be exactly what you might like. Do not always purchase the traditional black, navy and wine leotards instead of one of the more exciting fashion colors merely because you think those drab colors will somehow minimize the body. If you feel like wearing red—wear it. Wear whatever makes you happy that day.

Leg warmers, those tubes of knitted fabric that dancers wear to keep muscles relaxed, warm and flexible, are a fashion statement as well as a fitness aid. I love leg warmers. They are fun. They are so attractive and can also hide a less-than-perfect leg and ankle.

It is a good idea to consider a special aerobic shoe. Many regular athletic shoes are designed only for forward motion. Aerobics include many side movements. The tread of the sole should be designed to accommodate this sideways motion, and a strong heel support should prevent your foot from pronating.

Sweatbands are another fashion statement that is also practical. A headband can keep perspiration from running into your eyes.

If you are worried about looking heavy in the buttocks and stomach areas, perhaps you might choose a soft skirt or shorts to wear over the leotard.

You should have a track suit (you will find that you will be wearing this comfortable garment all the time) to wear over your exercise clothing while traveling to and from your place of exercise. The track suit should be loose and comfortable. It's a terrific sport outfit.

The body should be covered with layers of *light* clothing. If you are too cold, the muscles won't relax properly when you work out. You want your body temperature to regulate the heat and cold, not your clothing.

The Body Design by Gilda program works! Unlike some of the "miracle methods" I have seen.

In my search for physical fitness, I have tested everything. Being an optimist, I would consider every new weight-loss-and-inches-loss-made-fantastically-sim-

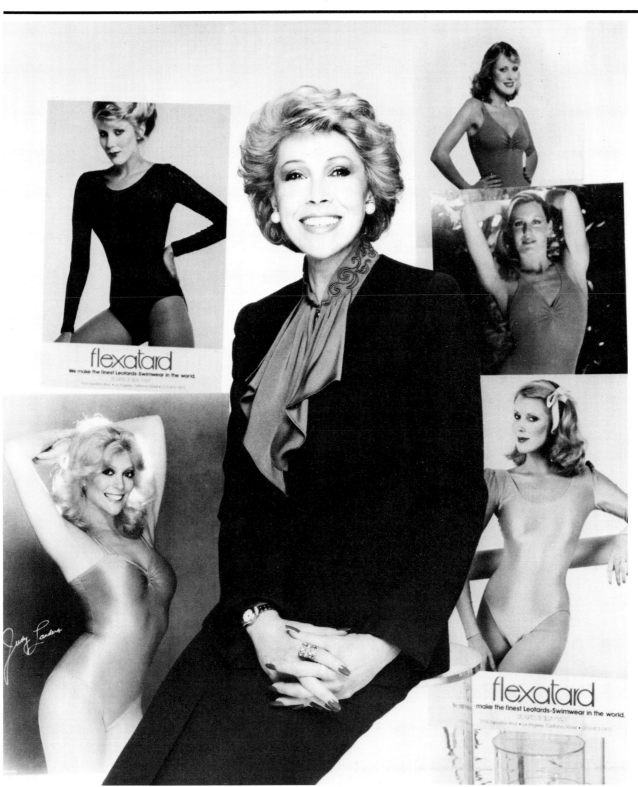

HARRY LANGDON

ple-in-mere-minutes miracle that came along. I ate grapes until fermentation set in. I have been jiggled, rubbed, salved and steamed.

I was even once gift-wrapped.

This happened a couple of years ago when a woman walked into my exercise studio, proclaiming, "I have a real miracle for your customers." Triumphantly, she placed a jar of the "miracle" glop on my desk and explained the process of figure wrapping.

I was curious . . . dangerously curious.

The idea was to rub this mayonnaise-like mess all over the body and then be wrapped, mummy-style, in plastic wrap and placed between two rubber sheets (or was it a rubber room?). After a half hour, the inches would just melt away.

"Hummm . . ." I said. "I wouldn't consider offering anything to my customers that I hadn't tested myself."

That was no problem for the body-wrap lady. She left a bottle of the miracle mayonnaise and complete instructions. I rushed home that evening, to experiment.

So there I was, standing naked in the bedroom, covered with mayonnaise and wrapped in Saran Wrap, when home comes my husband, Bob. My husband is the son of a Marx brother. As he stood in the doorway staring at me in my salad-dressing splendor, the heritage of Groucho, Gummo, Chico, Zeppo and Harpo came alive.

He raced to the kitchen and returned with a loaf of bread and a leer. "I think I am going to make a sandwich," he announced. Then he proceeded to clap my mayonnaise-soaked body between two pieces of bread.

At that moment I had no urge to be a sandwich. I attempted to distract the conversation away from what a person might consider my slightly humorous attire.

"This stuff is supposed to remove inches," I said pointedly, as I looked at my husband's waistline. "Take off your shirt."

Soon Bob's tummy was properly mayonnaised and Saran-Wrapped, and we started step two of the figure-wrapping procedure. This consisted of laying in a prone position for a quiet half hour, surrounded by rubber sheets, while the miracle mayonnaise transformed our bodies. Since we didn't have rubber sheets, we got onto the bed. We just had to lay quietly and think warm.

Unfortunately, the ceiling of the bedroom was mirrored. I detected a Marx giggle. Then a Marx grope. The body-wrap experiment ended very soon after that.

I never did offer body-wrapping to my students. Actually I have found that few of the gadgets and miracles are worth anything. Nothing works like regular exercise and common-sense eating habits to keep the body in great shape. Not only are most gimmicks a waste of money and time, many are actually dangerous.

The body-wrap advertising alleges that you can lose 4 to 12 inches with the first treatment. You can, but the loss is temporary, worthless and potentially harmful. Here's how it works: first you are wrapped in a mummylike fashion in tapes soaked in the magical solution (my at-home version was definitely a do-it-yourself method), and placed in a rubberized, airtight sweat suit or buried in the rubber sheets. This is to cut off air circulation. Next, you are told to relax for 30 to 60 minutes. Then the tapes are removed and the new figure is revealed.

There is a catch to this wonder.

The change is not permanent. In a few hours your startled body will revert back to its normal proportions. Worse yet, the antiperspirant action of the aluminum sulfate, the main ingredient in the magic solution, can produce a heat rash and the magnesium sulfate, another miracle ingredient, can cause skin irritation as well as a softening of the body tissues.

This gets worse.

The pressure of the tight bandages might reduce the blood volume in your extremities, diverting it to the internal organs and deeper body tissues. The whole process is nothing more than the body's reaction to dehydration and heat while wrapped in the sudden constriction of tissue and superficial blood vessels when exposed to cooler air. This is not only a waste of effort, time and money, but the results could actually be harmful.

There are many "miracles" that are not so miraculous.

Even more dangerous is a rubberized sweat suit. It is medically proven that permitting the body to overheat will produce dangerous conditions that occasionally have led to death. Uncontrolled sweating is unhealthy.

But these rubberized sweat suits are designed to make a person overperspire while, at the same time, retaining the maximum body heat.

These suits promise to promote rapid weight losses and, at first, the scales might seem to prove this promise to be true. You will be lighter immediately after hyper-sweating.

What you are losing is not fat. What is being lost is water, precious water. Water is something that you need in order to survive, and a rubberized sweat suit drains your body of its necessary fluids.

The weight loss is only temporary. The first glass of water taken after a period in the rubber suit will add the weight but not immediately refresh the drained body tissues.

Rubberized sweat suits rapidly wring the water from your body. They also trap the heat that radiates from your body and prevent the sweat from evaporating. The rubberized sweat suit interferes with nature's actual purpose for sweating, which is to cool the body.

If such unnatural sweating is permitted to continue with little or no evaporation, heat exhaustion, deep dehydration, exhaustion, and even heat stroke can occur.

Don't use the rubberized sweat suit.

Steam rooms offer some of the same drawbacks as the rubberized sweat suits. Certainly, I realize how popular steam rooms are. Every health club seems to have one. If every health club has a steam room, then they must be doing some good, you say, they must be safe.

Steam rooms can be badly misused.

The temperature inside a steam room is kept at about 130 degrees Fahrenheit and the humidity is kept very high. Again, you sweat profusely. But because of the high humidity, the sweat cannot evaporate to provide the natural cooling effect on the body. The result is that your body temperature rises to the same dangerous levels that are possible in the rubberized sweat suit. While the hot steam can cleanse your clogged pores, the possibility of overheating outweighs this slight advantage. *Avoid the steam room.*

Note: There is a difference between a sauna and a steam room. This important difference is that while the temperature inside a sauna goes as high as 185 degrees Fahrenheit, the humidity is kept very, very low. While you do sweat in a sauna, the perspiration evaporates quickly and the body is better able to regulate its internal temperature. While the steam room is potentially dangerous, the sauna is safe. But even a sauna does nothing to contribute to your overall physical fitness level. All it does is produce a relaxing effect.

The Jacuzzi—that super bathtub complete with hydro-massage units—has become a way of life for health-conscious Californians. Everyone seems to have a Jacuzzi. Social evenings are built around the Jacuzzi. Romances have flourished in the Jacuzzi.

While a Jacuzzi might be an interesting place for a party or an asset the morning after as a hangover cure, don't expect it to be a major contribution to any serious physical fitness program.

The hydro-massage unit is designed to direct high-pressure streams of water forcefully at the body, providing massage that can be gentle—or not so gentle. There have been claims that this action will help to redistribute fat.

This is just not possible. While the hydro-massage can bring a temporary relief to minor aches and help relax tensed muscles, it can't alter the composition of your body.

The hydro-massage is for fun and relaxation, not weight loss or fat redistribution.

While there are some social advantages to the hydro-massage, what I call "the vibrating junk" serves no purpose except to make the sellers of such gimmicks richer.

The vibrating belt is a perfect example of uselessness. Big promises are made by vibrating belt manufacturers. Just strap the belt around your waist, turn on the motor, and the belt jiggles away your spare tire. It does the work.

This is impossible. In order to lose weight or improve muscle tone, the body must expend energy. While the vibrating belt cannot do anything to help your body, it can actually tear and damage the very muscles you are attempting to strengthen. The only thing you will lose by purchasing a vibrating belt machine is from $200 to $600.

Now we get to pills, powders and magic formulas.

A lot has been said about prescribed diet pills. These high-powered uppers can cause a person to lose the urge to eat while stimulating the energy level. This can be dangerous (even while under a physician's care) because the pill taker can become so hyper that food is almost abandoned. The body becomes starved for nutrients and starts to feed on its own muscle. Uppers are also addictive, can cause a person to be unable to sleep, and change the personality. As the body addicts to these uppers, more and more pills are needed to produce the same results. Too many pills can kill. Of course, physicians recommend a person only use a controlled dosage for a short period of time, but many people want still more weight loss and take a few extra pills for a few days longer.

Prescribed diet pills can be dangerous.

While over-the-counter diet pills are not as dangerous as their high-power prescription cousins, they contain heavy doses of caffeine. You know, that stuff you try to avoid in coffee and soft drinks. Caffeine is a stimulant. It causes you to have more energy and suppresses the appetite—slightly. But everyday medical research finds more hazards involved with the consumption of caffeine, not the least of which is caffeine's tendency to give you a temporary lift that drops off suddenly, leaving you tired and irritable. The over-the-counter diet products are minimally effective and potentially dangerous.

New "miracles" come along every day. Starch blockers, those little pills that, when taken immediately before eating, prevented the body from absorbing limited quantities of starch, were a rage (at $25 a bottle) for a while. The safety of such innovations is often questionable. While starch blockers do prevent some starch from being added to your body weight, they have no effect on sugars, fats or proteins.

So long as there are people looking for the easy way to lose weight and become physically fit, dubious businessmen will be offering all manner of expensive—always expensive—wonders.

Some will produce limited results. Some will be useless. A few will actually be harmful. But the person who really wants to be fit forever cannot rely on gimmicks and fads. Pills that alter the body chemistry are only temporary. Proper eating and nutrition habits, coupled with regular exercise, can alter the body's chemistry and physiology for life.

The best piece of exercise equipment you have is your own mind and mental attitude. No machine or gadget alone can make you succeed in making those wonderful changes in your body. You must make yourself succeed.

It takes a tremendous amount of self-motivation to stay on any challenging physical improvement program. This kind of commitment is difficult to maintain. Phones ring. Children demand attention. There are always emergencies. There is so much with which to cope. But keep telling yourself:

"I want to do this for myself. I will not be deterred by the demands and problems of life. When I am more fit, I will be better able to handle these demands. I will be stronger. I will be more attractive. I will have more energy. Everything is getting better. I must keep exercising."

Promise me you will keep telling yourself that. And, in turn, I will make some promises to you. I promise that those of you who will take the Body Design by Gilda program and make it a part of your life . . . I promise that if you follow the program every other day for three to six months, you will develop a sense of well-being and will like yourself more . . . I promise that you will look better . . . and I promise that you will want to continue the program for the rest of your wonderful energy-filled life.

Now comes the warning that you have all heard before but it is so very important. It is imperative that before beginning any exercise program that you become completely aware of your physical condition. If you have not seen a physician in the last six months, please do so. If you have any history of heart problems, high blood pressure, neck, shoulder or back problems, or problems with your feet, please discuss it with your doctor. It is so important that you be aware of your health before starting the program.

CHAPTER 7
THE BODY DESIGN BY GILDA PROGRAM

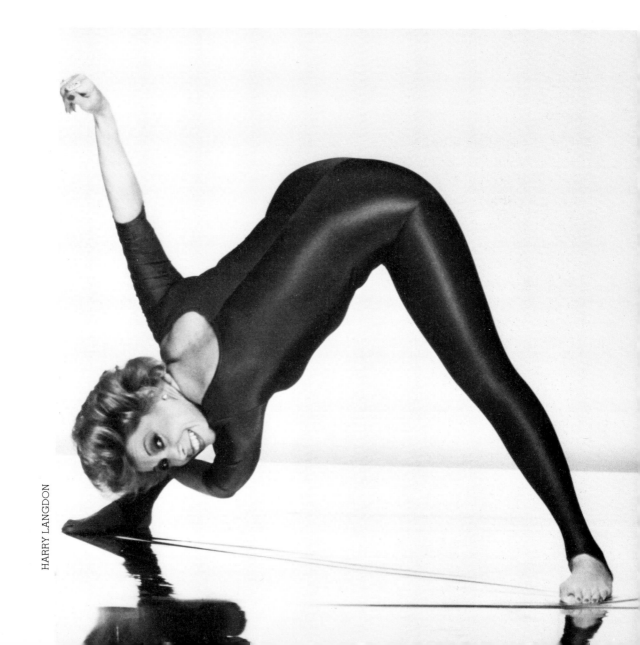

HARRY LANGDON

POSTURE

Happy the man who could
search out the cause of things.

—VIRGIL

So far, I have been telling you that it will take time to change that fat into muscle. I have been telling you that nothing happens overnight. I have been telling you not to expect immediate changes.

Now I am going to tell you something quite different.

By improving your posture, you often will see immediate results. The waist will seem slimmer. The breasts will be more shapely. You appear to be taller and sleeker. All this can happen merely by correcting bad posture.

Most of us have poor posture.

You see people walking down the street with heads thrust forward as if in a race with their torsos. You see people slumped in chairs forcing the backs to curve in awkward and unhealthful positions. You see people with sagging and defeated-looking shoulders and double chins. And, of course, you see people with protruding stomachs.

Correct posture is extremely important to be ultimately successful in the Body Design by Gilda program. You must stand straight with the body in proper alignment. If you exercise with poor posture, you will be training your muscles incorrectly. This is very damaging. The muscles will not be strengthened in the correct form. The body will then adapt to the stress of the incorrect positioning.

These are the visible manifestations of poor posture, but often what we do not see is the damage done to the inner muscle structure by poor posture.

Such as:

—If you are dizzy or suffer neck, shoulder and arm pains, this
could be the result of a forward head.

—If you have back or neck strain, this might just be caused by those stooped shoulders.

—If there is a tightness in the muscles of the chest that is affecting the performance of the lungs (and sometimes the heart muscle), this is often traceable to poor overall posture.

—If your circulation is poor, if menstruation is painful, if you have ruptured discs, if you have backaches, this is quite often caused by a protruding abdomen and lumbar lordosis (swayback).

—If you have poor blood circulation, sometimes the cause is hyperextended knees.

Poor posture, even if only one part of the body suffers from a posture defect, increases the strain on muscles, ligaments and joints throughout the body.

To check your posture, I recommend the Plumb Bob Test. Start by looking at yourself sideways in the mirror. Imagine a plumb line hung from the ceiling to the floor. The vertical line of the imaginary string should run through your ear, through the tip of the shoulder, through the very center of the hipbone and slightly to the front of the center of the knee and the anklebone.

Proper posture is important because it helps to minimize the stress on the body. If you hold your head back and over the shoulders, the weight of the head will be correctly transmitted through the neck to the back. This is the positioning your body was created to have to make the most functional use of the muscle and bone structure.

Good posture begins with the head. Move your chin back, tuck it in so your ear does align over your shoulder. Pull the chest up as if a string from your breastbone is lifting your chest up and out. Your shoulders will then assume a relaxed backward position in correct alignment. Pull the stomach in as you tuck the buttocks under your trunk. Lengthen the trunk by standing erect. Look impressive and well balanced. Keep knees slightly relaxed, not locked out. Keep your weight evenly distributed between the front and back of your feet.

A person who has proper posture immediately looks more fit than a person who permits the body to sag and droop. Good posture puts the minimum amount of physical demands on the muscle structure and redistributes the body weight on the skeletal structure where nature intended it to be. Improper posture causes the muscles to deform in a strained effort to hold the body erect.

An important part of good posture is proper breathing.

Always remember to breathe deeply through the nostrils and exhale through the mouth. Keep taking in that oxygen that feeds the blood and muscles. Proper breathing will enable you to keep exercising longer and perform more exercise repetitions. Sometimes people forget to breathe while exercising. This produces a smothering effect and can cause dizziness and headaches.

A couple of exercises can help you to learn how to breathe deeply from the diaphragm, a muscle under the lungs.

1. Place your hand just below the rib cage so that you can feel the diaphragm muscle expanding and contracting. Inhale through the nose. Now blow out all the air from your lungs. Without letting go of your chest, slowly begin to sip in air as if you were sipping it with a straw. Hold that breath, then release. The diaphragm muscles should expand as you breathe in and contract when you exhale. Repeat this exercise five times.

2. Next blow out all the air from your lungs and take five little sips of air. Count to five and then release the air in five small separate puffs. Repeat this exercise five times.

Spend 10 to 15 minutes a day doing breathing exercises. Yes, you will have time. Do them while you are waiting for a bus or driving to work or waiting in line at the grocery store. Do some high-quality breathing.

Improved posture and breathing produce immediate results. Most students leave the first class with added bounce to the step. They walk with confident strides, heads erect and alert, and shoulders squared and back. If there is such a thing as an instant method for a more handsome/beautiful you, that method would be becoming aware of the benefits of proper posture.

A Gilda Rule: Head Back! Chin in! Chest Out! Shoulders Relaxed! Stomach in! Buttocks Tucked! Watch That Posture.

THE EXERCISE

THE POSTURE CHECK

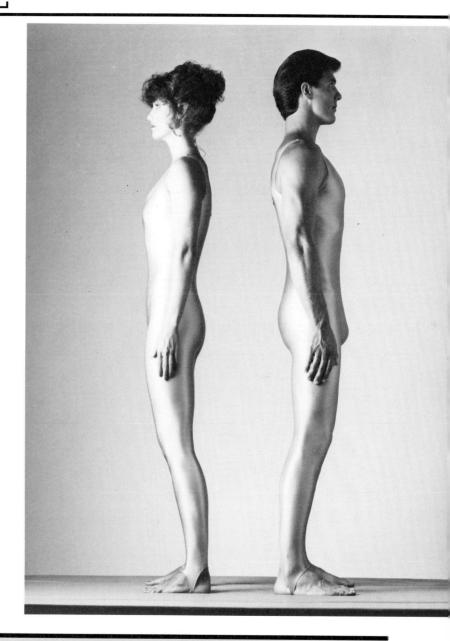

1 Stand with feet approximately hip width apart, toes pointing forward. Knees should be relaxed, buttocks slightly tight, stomach pressed in, back erect, shoulders relaxed, chin tucked in so ears are in line over shoulders.

2 Practice this against a wall.

3 Practice it at least once a day.

BENEFITS:	Improves the posture and places the weight on the skeletal structure in proper alignment.
CAUTION:	Keep chin in. Maintain proper body alignment. Keep weight evenly distributed between front and back. Pull the arches up slightly.

WARM-UP STRETCHING

Now start to turn on!

A proper warm-up period is important to stretch and elongate the muscles. This helps to avoid injury. When you first start to exercise, the muscles are tight. They need to be carefully loosened and stretched so that later in the exercise program when the exercises become more demanding, the muscles will not strain.

An important part of the warm-up is increasing the body temperature. That is why it is called a "warm-up." By beginning the exercise session at a lower intensity than you plan to work during the training portions of the program, your muscles slowly begin to work while at the same time they produce heat.

Why is this heat so important?

The working muscles heat the blood that passes through them which in turn increases the heat of the entire body. When blood vessels are heated, they open wider to supply more blood to the muscles. This temperature increase steps up the functioning of the heart and lungs, improving their ability to handle the demands of exercising.

The aerobic enzymes within the muscles increase as a result of activity and energy production becomes more efficient. This helps to burn unnecessary fat. The fluids of the joints and the lubricating fluids of the tendons are heated and become less viscous. This makes movement easier and helps to prevent possible muscle injury.

For the first 30 minutes of the Body Design by Gilda program, you are not only exercising but you are very carefully warming and stretching every muscle in the body. Each exercise is carefully designed and placed to lead to the next exercise.

The program is meant to be learned as a series of routine movements. At first, the program might seem complicated. It is! You will have to work.

Keep trying!

I understand that the Body Design by Gilda program can be challenging, even for the frequent exerciser. If, at first, you cannot do every exercise, don't worry.

While some of my students can do the entire Body Design by Gilda program immediately, I have designed the Four Week to Success System for acclimating your muscles to exercising.

Do the program a minimum of three times a week. Each week, you will do *some* of the exercises until you are limber enough and the cardiovascular system is improved enough to be able to complete the entire Body Design by Gilda program.

It will happen fast!

The improvement comes so fast; one day you may only be able to complete a few repetitions of a particularly difficult exercise, but several days later, you might be elated to find that you are breezing through the required repetitions.

Don't feel badly if you do have some difficulty with a few of these exercises. I have seen famous athletes and movie stars with fabulous bodies struggling with an exercise that is using a previously neglected muscle group.

Just keep trying . . . you can do it! Now, put on some of your favorite fast music and start getting that body *hot.*

THE EXERCISE
SHOULDER ROLLS

1 Relax arms to side.

2 Move the shoulders back, up and forward in a smooth, circular motion.

3 Do motion forward eight times.

4 Reverse the motion eight times.

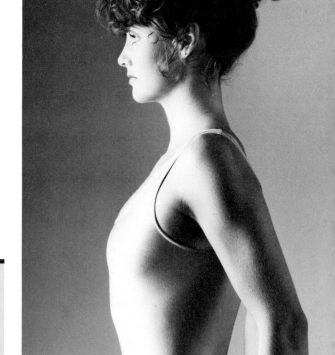

BENEFITS: Releases tension in the shoulders and prepares the muscles for stretching.
Muscles involved: Deltoids, upper trapezius.

POSTURE: Basic posture position (plumb line).

CAUTION: Keep relaxed. Do not tense muscles.
Make sure the shoulders are doing the movement and not the arms.
Keep chin pulled in.

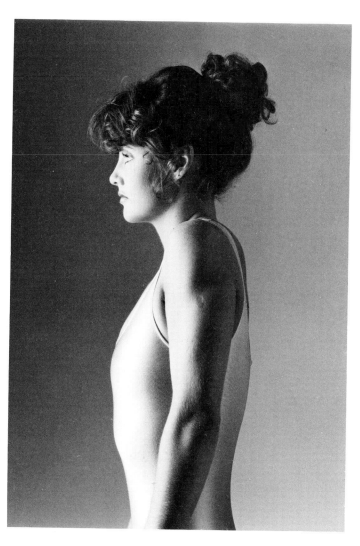

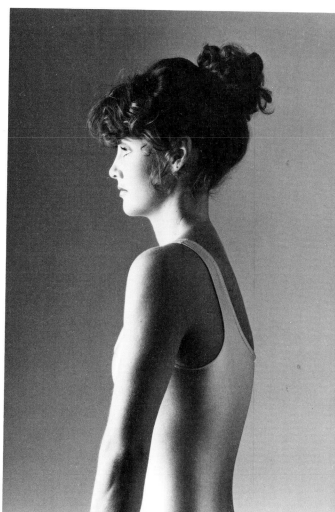

THE EXERCISE

DEEP BREATHING

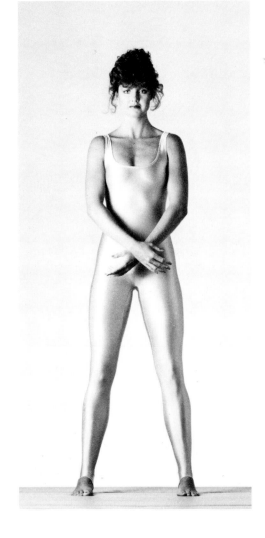
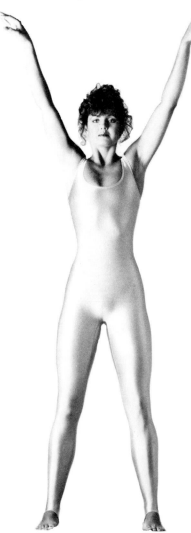

1 Stand with feet approximately hip width apart, toes pointing forward. Knees should be relaxed, buttocks tucked under, stomach pressed in, back erect, shoulders relaxed.

2 Inhale deeply, bringing the arms out to the side and up over the head.

3 Exhale very slowly through the mouth. Return the arms gracefully down next to your sides. Repeat four times.

BENEFITS: Improves breathing habits.

THE EXERCISE
ARM CIRCLES

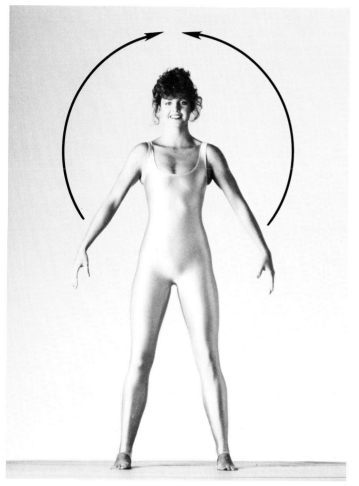

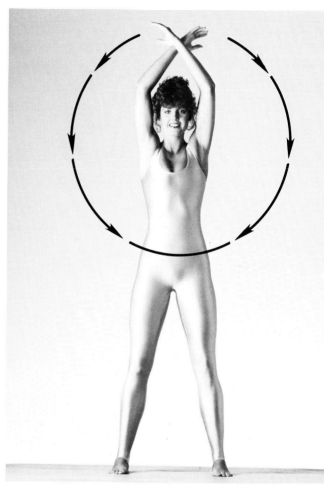

1 Extend arms to the sides.

2 Move arms in a circular motion crossing at the center of the body.

3 Do eight circles clockwise and eight counterclockwise.

BENEFITS:	Raises the temperature within the muscles of the arms, shoulders and upper back. Muscles involved: Deltoids, trapezius, rotor cuff muscles, pectorals.
POSTURE:	Basic posture position. Keep chin in.
CAUTION:	Keep the body stabilized, moving only the arms.

THE EXERCISE
STRETCH MEDLEY I

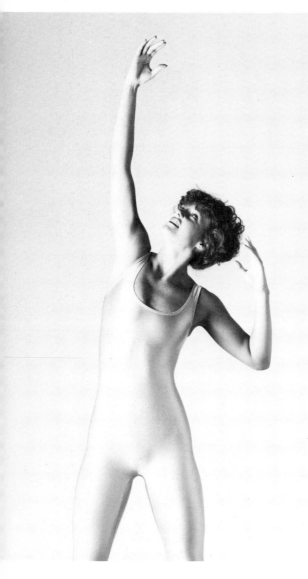

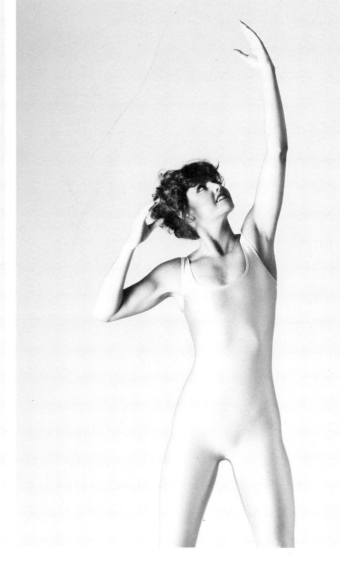

1 Start with feet shoulder width apart.

2 Alternately stretch arms overhead, stretching from the rib cage.

3 Repeat eight times.

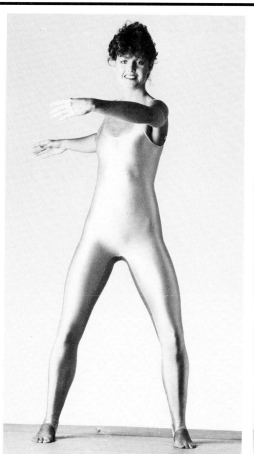
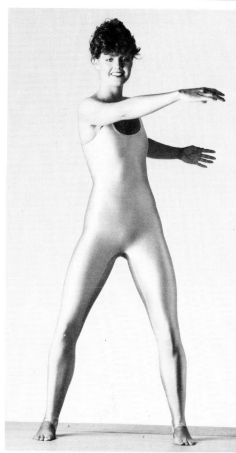

4 With arms slightly curved and extended at shoulder level, twist side to side from the waist, keeping the knees bent and the hips stable.

5 Repeat eight times.

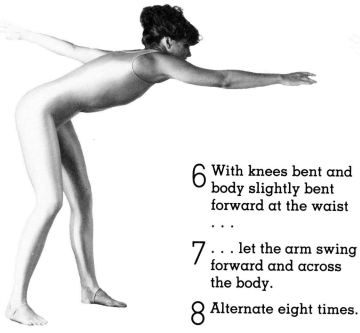

6 With knees bent and body slightly bent forward at the waist . . .

7 . . . let the arm swing forward and across the body.

8 Alternate eight times.

STRETCH MEDLEY I

9 Bend torso all the way down.

10 Loosely swing arms from side to side.

11 Repeat eight times. Remain in forward position and continue to next exercise.

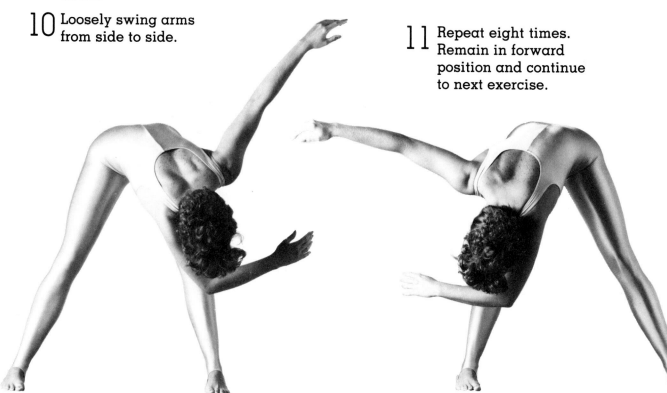

BENEFITS: Stretches and warms up arms, waist, back and legs without overtaxing the body. Muscles involved: Latissimus dorsi, lower and mid-back, buttocks and hamstrings.

POSTURE: Be sure to keep knees bent and hips stable when you roll up.

CAUTION: Straight legs could put unnecessary strain on lower back when bending forward. Do not go to full range of movement on first set.

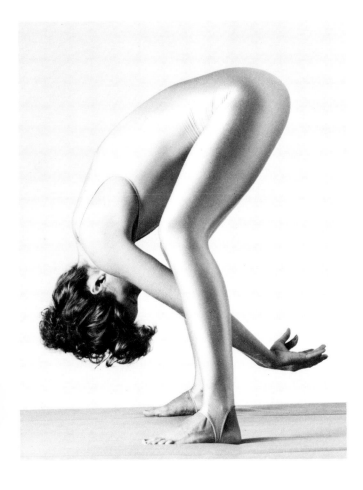

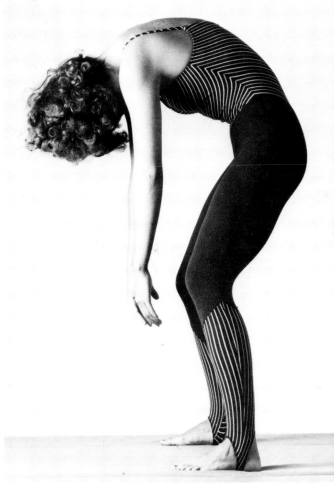

1 While still bent over, reach the hands through the legs while keeping the knees bent.

2 Reach through for eight counts in a small range of motion.

3 Roll body up.

BENEFITS:	Stretches the back and the muscles in the back of the leg. Muscles involved: Back and hamstrings.
POSTURE:	Keep those knees bent, relax head and neck.
CAUTION:	Do not force or bounce upper body while reaching through the legs.

THE EXERCISE
STRETCH MEDLEY II

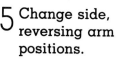

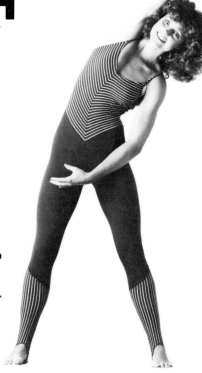

1 Return to erect position.

2 Reach one arm over head, causing waist to bend.

3 Other arm reaches low across waist in opposition.

4 Reach for eight counts in the extended position.

5 Change side, reversing arm positions.

6 Reach for eight counts.

9 Drop upper body further toward floor.

10 Place hands behind head with elbows out to the side.

11 Hang for eight counts.

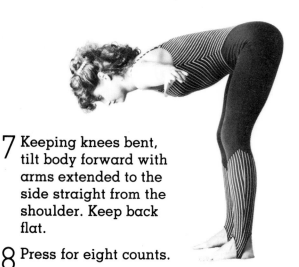

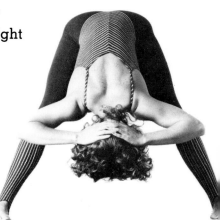

7 Keeping knees bent, tilt body forward with arms extended to the side straight from the shoulder. Keep back flat.

8 Press for eight counts.

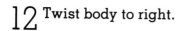

12 Twist body to right.

13 Place left hand on right ankle.

14 Stretch right hand toward ceiling, gently pull the upper body toward leg.

15 Hold for eight counts.

16 Change arms to other side.

17 Hold for eight counts.

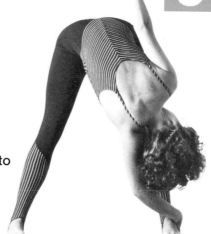

18 Reach through the center of legs for eight counts, keeping knees bent.

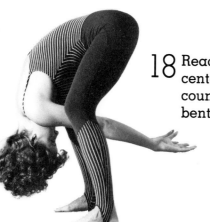

19 Return to erect position. Place hands on hips, tighten buttock muscles and move pelvis forward.

20 Do small tucks eight times.

21 Repeat entire exercise; counts in eights, fours, twos and ones.

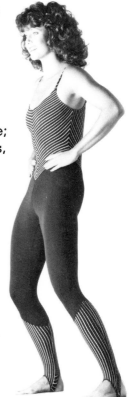

BENEFITS: This is a complete body warm-up with emphasis on back and hamstring stretching.
Muscles involved: Back and hamstrings.

POSTURE: Be sure to keep the knees slightly bent, and the abdominals held in.

CAUTION: Do not go to full range of movement until second time through. Keep movements controlled. Do not bounce.

THE EXERCISE
LEG SQUAT

1 With knees bent and placed directly over toes, hang body forward and place hands on floor.

2 With heels on floor, press hips down for a count of five.

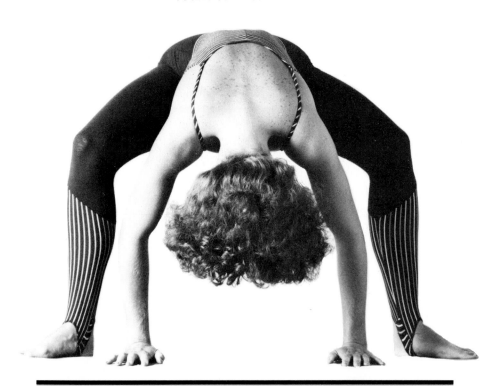

BENEFITS: Warms up the front of thighs and inner thighs, stretches hamstrings.
Muscles involved: Quadriceps, adductors and hamstrings.

POSTURE: Keep knees over toes.

CAUTION: Do not bounce; do not overstretch.

THE EXERCISE
SIDE LUNGE

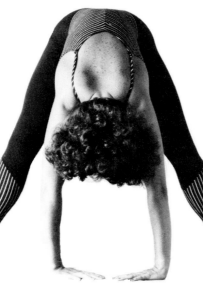

1 From the squat position, straighten legs, place hands on the floor with hands and fingers turned inward.

2 Turn toes outward toward the side.

3 Bend at the right knee.

4 Press gently toward the right leg stretching inner thigh muscles.

5 Carefully go to left side.

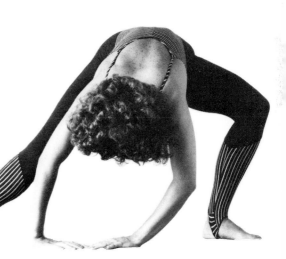

6 Repeat two sets of four, two sets of two.

BENEFITS:	Stretches the inner thigh. Increases flexibility. Muscle involved: Adductor.
POSTURE:	Keep knees over toes and feet flat on ground.
CAUTION:	Gradually increase the range of movement. Do not do full range until the sets of two. Never bend knee more than 90 degrees.

THE EXERCISE
ROAD
RUNNER

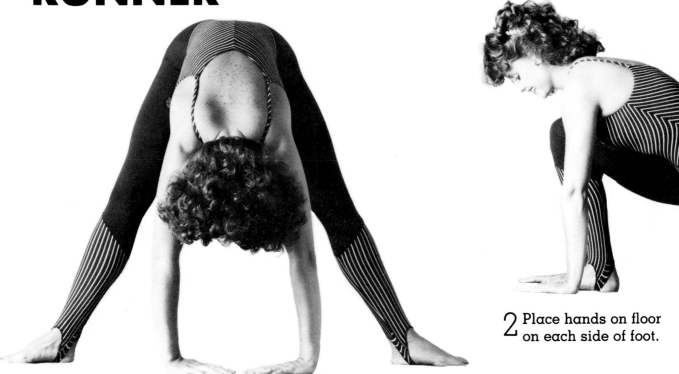

2 Place hands on floor on each side of foot.

1 From the lunge position, straighten both legs and rotate body to one side.

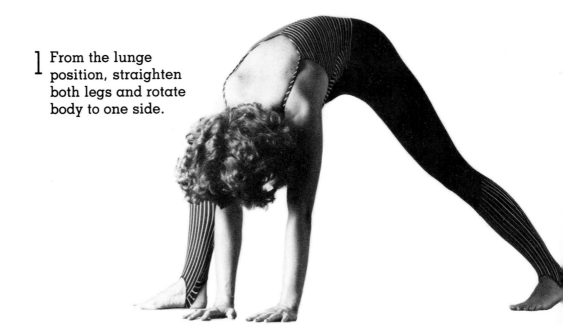

3 Bend the front leg to a 90-degree angle and straighten back leg with feet parallel and hips even and squared toward floor. With head and neck relaxed, deepen position for eight counts.

4 Keeping feet in same position, attempt to carefully straighten the front leg.

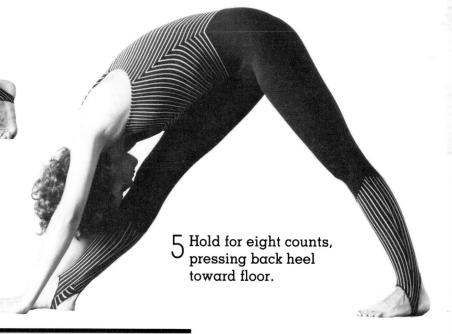

5 Hold for eight counts, pressing back heel toward floor.

BENEFITS: Stretches the back and front of thigh, hip and inner thigh.
Muscles involved: Hip flexor (iliopsoas), upper hamstring and buttocks.

POSTURE: Keep the heel and knee of the front leg in a straight vertical line with the shoulder.

CAUTION: This is a challenging exercise. Keep front heel on floor at all times (if the heel rises the foot is too close to the body).

6 Repeat in one set of four and one set of two.

7 Repeat entire series on other side.

THE EXERCISE
HEEL LIFTS

1 Walk hands to center. With feet apart and legs straight, walk hands forward away from body to a comfortable range. In this position lift heels eight times. With heels lifted, hold for eight counts.

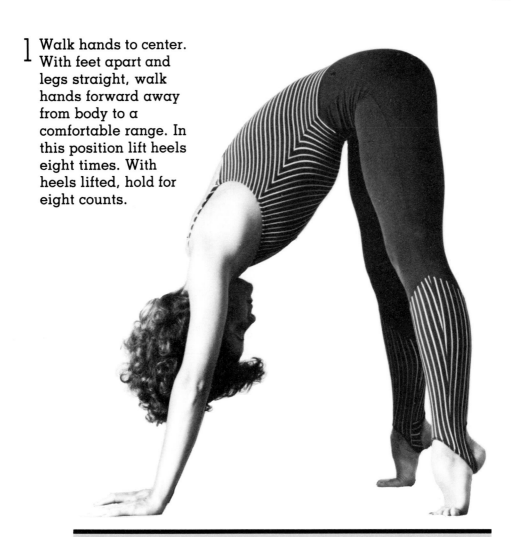

BENEFITS: Stretches and warms calves, hamstrings, shoulders and upper back.
Muscles involved: Calves, hamstrings, shoulders and upper back.

CAUTION: Do not arch the back or lift the head.
Keep ears next to arms.

THE EXERCISE
TOE-TO-HEEL ROCK

1 From the last heel-lift position, walk hands closer to body. Lower heels.

2 With legs shoulder width apart, knees slightly bent, walk feet together.

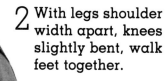

4 Shift weight to heels, and lift toes off the floor.

3 Placing weight on toes, lift heels off floor.

5 Do eight times.

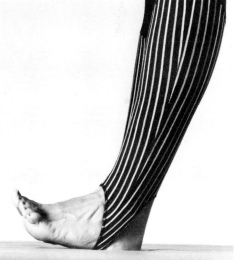

BENEFITS: Works calves—front and back, all muscles in the foot, and stretches hamstrings, buttocks and lower back.
Muscles involved: Calves, foot musculature, hamstrings, buttocks and lower back.

THE EXERCISE
HIP STRETCH

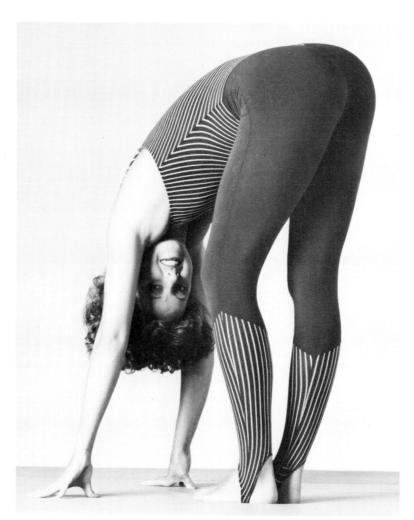

1 With feet together (legs straight) and hands as close to floor as possible, bend one leg at a time until you feel a stretch in the hip.

2 Alternate legs for a count of sixteen.

BENEFITS:	Stretches back of thighs and hips. Muscles involved: Hamstrings and buttocks.
POSTURE:	Keep the upper body relaxed. Keep heels pressed into floor.
CAUTION:	Do not snap (hyperextend) the knees. Do not force the knees.

AEROBICS

Now you really get hot!

The word "aerobic" means living or active only in the presence of oxygen. The purpose of aerobic exercise is to improve and strengthen the cardiovascular system: the heart, the lungs and the blood vessels. This was the reason that actress and model Maud Adams took the Body Design by Gilda program. She is one of those very fortunate persons who has never had a weight problem. She is tall with long and lean legs. She is naturally perfectly proportioned.

So why did Maud Adams need the program?

She wanted to improve the way she felt. She wanted to have plenty of energy to meet the demands of her hectic schedule. She wanted her important internal organs and muscles to be in just as great condition as her outer body.

Aerobics help the body to function more efficiently. Through aerobic training, the body is better able to take oxygen from the air and deliver it to all the internal muscles and organs that utilize it to create energy and perform work.

Aerobics speed you up!

An important benefit of aerobic training is that it will transform the body into a more efficient calorie-burning machine. Aerobic exercises and the metabolic changes that are the result of aerobic exercises cause the body to burn fat stored in the muscle. This increases the muscle part of that crucial fat-to-muscle ratio. By exercising your muscles at a level that causes your heart rate to reach a level of 70 to 85 percent of the maximum beats per minute, you unleash the benefits of aerobics and strengthen the heart muscle.

The term aerobic exercise has replaced the term cardiovascular exercise for good reason. While it is true that this form of exercise improves the function of the heart and blood vessels as indicated by the old term "cardiovascular," the effects of aerobic exercise on the larger body muscles are much greater and more important for fat loss. Aerobic training makes the skeletal muscles efficient factories for utilizing oxygen and fat in relatively large amounts to make energy. The increased energy production allows us to do more work and make it feel easy.

Monitoring the heart rate during aerobics has been an effective way to gain more knowledge of how our bodies respond to the conditioning programs we put them through. It is important for you to be familiar with your own *resting* and *training* (target) heart rates, so that you will be aware of how hard you are and should be working. This is all part of a safe aerobic program.

The easiest and most accurate way to determine your *resting* heart rate is to take your pulse first thing in the morning, before you get out of bed.

1. Gently place your index and middle fingers on your *carotid artery*, which is found in the neck; or on your *radial artery*, which is found on the thumb side of your wrist, to locate your pulse.
2. Count your heartbeats for ten seconds.
3. Multiply that number by six.

The number you will get will be your *resting* heart rate. As your cardiovascular fitness increases, your *resting* heart rate will decrease to a slower rate. Use your *resting* heart rate as a measure of your long-term fitness improvement.

To get the optimum benefit from an aerobic program, you must train at a specific level of intensity. To calculate what level is right for you (your training heart rate), you must first determine your maximum heart rate. This is done by subtracting your age from 220. This is your theoretical maximum heart rate. Your training heart should be 70 to 85 percent of this number.

To determine your *training* heart rate, immediately upon completion of the most strenuous segment of your aerobic workout, take the following steps:

1. Find your pulse using the same procedure as step 1 above.
2. Count for only six seconds (your pulse returns to the *resting* level very quickly).
3. Multiply that number by ten.

The number you get will be your *training* heart rate. UNDER NO CIRCUM-STANCES SHOULD THIS NUMBER EXCEED THE MAXIMUM HEART RATE LISTED IN THE CHART ON THE FACING PAGE for your age.

Using the "Target Zone Chart":

After you have determined your *training* heart rate, look at the Target Zone Chart (below) according to your age. If your *training* heart rate exceeds the highest number of your "target heart range," SLOW DOWN. If the number you get is below the lowest number of your "target heart range," WORK HARDER! By using this chart you can get a better idea of the proper range you should be working within.

Target Zone Chart
(Age Adjusted Heart Rate Chart)

Age	Maximum Heart Rate	Target Heart Rate	Target Heart Rate Range
20	200	150	140–170
25	195	146	137–166
30	190	142	133–162
35	185	139	130–157
40	180	135	126–153
45	175	131	123–149
50	170	127	119–145
55	165	124	116–140
60	160	120	112–136
65	155	116	109–132

Approach aerobics sensibly and realistically. If you cannot walk up a flight of stairs without finding yourself out of breath, this is a definite indication that your body needs an aerobic tune-up.

Aerobic exercises will tune the body.

Be cautious when you start an aerobic program. Don't push yourself too hard. At least, don't overpush yourself at first. If you can only accomplish two minutes of the aerobic portion of the program in the beginning, keep working until you can do those two minutes comfortably. Then try for five minutes.

Your body will improve quickly. Soon you will be able to do ten minutes of the aerobic choreography with the proper awareness of elevating that heart rate and pumping that fat-burning oxygen to those muscles.

Keep looking toward the future. As your body strengthens . . . after three months . . . six months . . . a year . . . you will be comfortably able to accomplish the full 20 minutes of the aerobics program. At first, this might seem so very difficult. But you will improve. You will be able to do the program. Keep working. Hundreds of thousands of people have had to go through the same struggle to succeed that you are now facing. And they did succeed.

A fit person is a person who is able to exercise vigorously and recover quickly. Technically, this means that the heart rate should decrease by at least 30 beats per minute during the 30-second period after the completion of a strenuous exercise session of two minutes or more. Aerobics give your heart the capability to meet the heaviest demands and still function efficiently.

Remember: During aerobics, your toe should hit the ground first, then the ball of your foot, and then your heel. This is very important to avoid injury.

Now breathe deeply through the nose and out the mouth. Turn up that music. Get ready to dance toward success.

THE EXERCISE
PRANCING

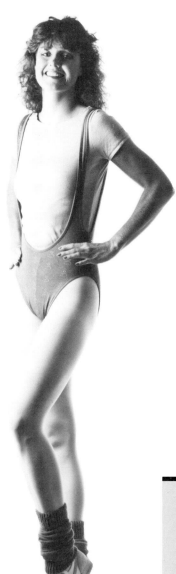

1 Place feet parallel and hands on hips.

2 Lift the knees alternately.

3 As the foot comes down, press it into the floor—toe first, then the ball of the foot, then the heel.

4 Do with a light, springing action.

TIME:	60 seconds.
BENEFITS:	Begins aerobic exercise, slowly starts to increase the heart rate.
POSTURE:	Upper torso and head should be erect.
CAUTION:	With all the running in place exercises it is most important that the foot making contact with the floor touches down on the ball of the foot first and then descends to make full heel contact. This is important for proper shock absorption and the prevention of shin splints.

THE EXERCISE
LITTLE JOG IN PLACE

1 Continue the prance but begin to lift the heel and knees slightly higher.

2 Swing both arms parallel overhead from side to side.

TIME:	60 seconds.
BENEFITS:	Begins to gradually increase the heart rate.
POSTURE:	Upper torso and head should be erect.
CAUTION:	Be sure to press heels into the floor each time. Keep the knees lifted in front of the body.

THE EXERCISE
KNEE-UPS

1 With feet hip width apart . . .

2 . . . lift knees even higher.

3 Lift arms straight up to ceiling. . .

4 . . . pulling elbows down toward floor.

TIME:	30 seconds.
POSTURE:	Upper torso and head should be erect.
CAUTION:	Keep the shoulders relaxed. Work the arms, not the shoulders. Keep pressing the heels into the floor.

SIDE KICKS

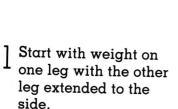

1 Start with weight on one leg with the other leg extended to the side.

2 Raise arm opposite the extended leg to form a straight line.

3 Change sides with a swinging, pendulum, feeling, with lowered hand tapping thigh.

TIME:	30 seconds.
POSTURE:	Keep the chest lifted. Do not lean forward.
CAUTION:	Do not stop the movements. Start with a smaller movement and work up to a greater range of motion. Keep head centered.

FRONT KICKS

1 Keep body erect with weight centered.

2 Hop from one leg to the other with legs kicking straight out in front of body.

3 With arms bent, reach straight overhead.

TIME:	30 seconds.
BENEFITS:	Further challenges balance and coordination.
POSTURE:	Keep weight evenly distributed between both legs.
CAUTION:	Do not lean back. Progress slowly to greater ranges of forward leg motions.

THE EXERCISE
BACK KICKS

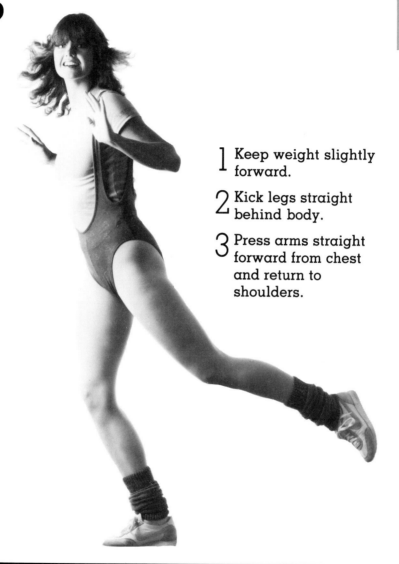

1 Keep weight slightly forward.

2 Kick legs straight behind body.

3 Press arms straight forward from chest and return to shoulders.

TIME: 30 seconds.

BENEFITS: Works arms, buttocks, chest and calf muscles.

POSTURE: Lean forward and keep a small amount of stomach tension.

CAUTION: Be sure the heels press into the floor when they land.

THE EXERCISE
FORWARD LUNGES

1 Start with one leg bent and lunged forward while other leg is straight to the back.

2 Jump and reverse positions of legs.

3 Arms are straight with one extended overhead and the other straight ahead moving in a hammering action.

TIME:	30 seconds.
BENEFITS:	This is one of the more challenging exercises that works all the leg and hip muscles.
POSTURE:	Keep the back straight, the upper body erect, and the shoulders relaxed. Keep some stomach tension.
CAUTION:	Try to keep legs parallel, with the foot pointing directly ahead.

THE EXERCISE
LEGS
APART

Same exercise as the forward lunge, but the stance is widened.

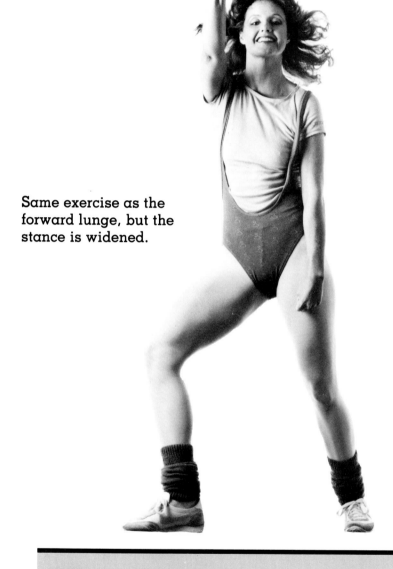

TIME:	30 seconds.
BENEFITS:	Puts more demands on the outer and inner hip and thigh area.
POSTURE:	Same as with the forward lunges.
CAUTION:	Do not permit the knees to twist.

THE EXERCISE
JUMPING JACKS

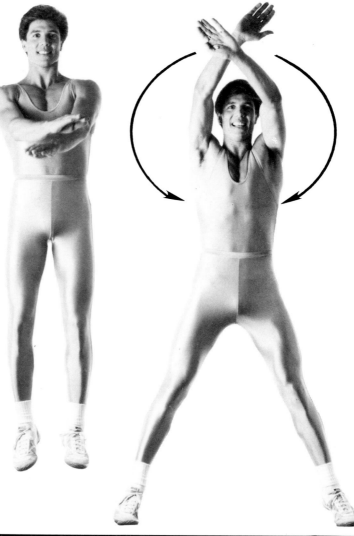

1 Start with feet together.

2 In a jumping motion, separate feet to the side.

3 Move arms in a full circle in front of the body.

TIME:	30 seconds.
BENEFITS:	Keeps the heart beating at a peak rate. Works shoulders, chest and upper back as well as leg and hip muscles.
POSTURE:	The chest should be lifted and the back kept straight. Keep chin in.
CAUTION:	Keep movements smooth and even.

THE EXERCISE
CHORUS KICKS

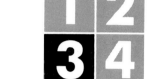

1 Place weight on one leg while lifting other leg toward chest (with knee bent) and hop. Keep arms straight out to side.

2 Return to starting position with a jump.

3 Kick same leg straight out to waist height with another hop.

4 Return leg with a jump.

5 Alternate legs.

TIME: 30 seconds.

POSTURE: Keep the chest up and shoulders squared.

CAUTION: Do not allow body to tip forward as leg lifts. Start out low and go higher as your flexibility increases.

BENEFITS: Same as others but with more work for the hip flexors (iliopsoas), a somewhat larger muscle group.

THE EXERCISE
CHORUS KICKS WITH ARMS

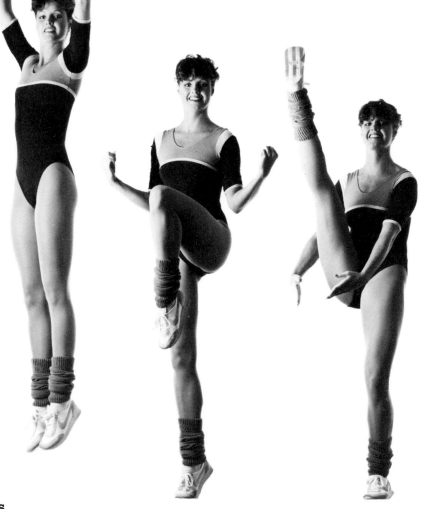

1 Same as chorus kicks only arms pull from overhead as knee bends.

2 Arms lower and clap under leg as leg extends.

TIME	30 seconds.
BENEFITS:	This is an important coordination movement that is great for the hips, thighs and shoulders.
POSTURE:	Keep the chest up and shoulders squared.

STRAIGHT KICKS

1 Kick legs straight to the front to waist level with a hopping motion.

2 With arms straight, swing arms overhead with opposite hand touching opposite toe.

TIME:	30 seconds.
BENEFITS:	This is the most demanding of the aerobic exercises. The heart rate should be at its highest.
POSTURE:	Keep upper torso erect and legs straight.
CAUTION:	Lift leg only as high as you can without bending the knee or straining your back.

THE EXERCISE
ALTERNATING SIDE LUNGE

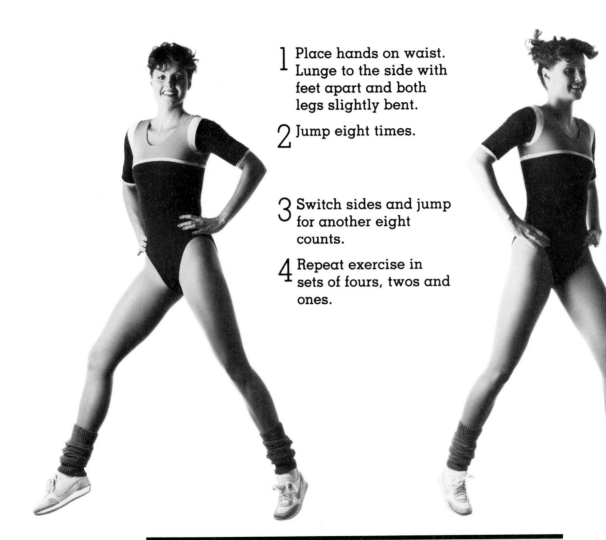

1 Place hands on waist. Lunge to the side with feet apart and both legs slightly bent.

2 Jump eight times.

3 Switch sides and jump for another eight counts.

4 Repeat exercise in sets of fours, twos and ones.

TIME: 60 seconds.

BENEFITS: Maintains heart rate.

POSTURE: The front leg should be slightly more bent than the back leg. Be sure to make heel contact with each step.

THE EXERCISE
STEP-LIFTING FORWARD

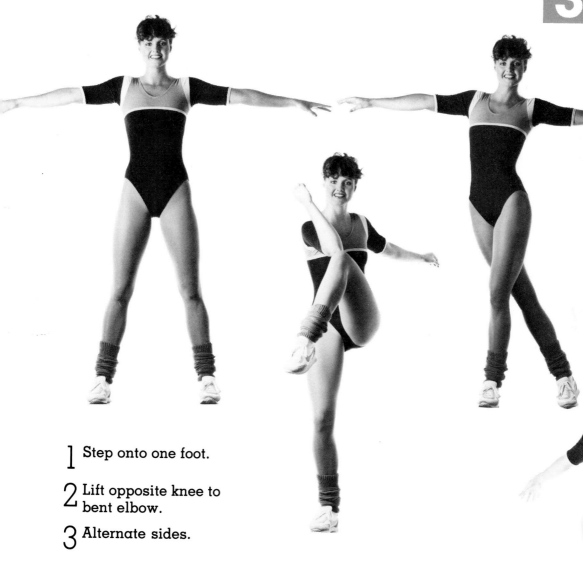

1 Step onto one foot.

2 Lift opposite knee to bent elbow.

3 Alternate sides.

TIME:	75 seconds.
BENEFITS:	Gradually lowers the heart rate. Works the waist.
POSTURE:	Keep chest lifted. Do not bend forward.

THE EXERCISE
STEP-LIFTING SIDE

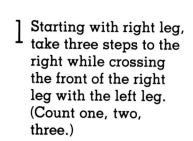

1 Starting with right leg, take three steps to the right while crossing the front of the right leg with the left leg. (Count one, two, three.)

2 On the fourth count, lift knee to elbow as in previous exercise.

3 Repeat on other side.

TIME:	75 seconds.
BENEFITS:	Lowers heart rate gradually.
POSTURE:	Keep chest lifted.
CAUTION:	Watch your balance.

UPPER BACK, ARMS AND CHEST

The muscles of the upper body are all interrelated. It is important to condition these muscles so that the body develops the strength to hold itself in correct posture. Of primary importance are the muscles of the upper back, which need to be strengthened to give the body an upright appearance. When these muscles are weak, the back has a tendency to sag and the shoulders become rounded.

It is important to develop the arm muscles, not only for a better apppearance but to give the arms strength to function better. If the arms are strong for lifting, pressure is removed from the back. The stronger the arms are, the more you can use them. The more the arms are used, the more calories are burned. The more calories you burn—the more fat you lose. A simple cycle!

If you want to build more muscle mass while doing the arm series, you need to add more resistance—weights. Attaching three to five round weights to the wrists is usually enough resistance to add muscle mass to the arms.

All these exercises not only help develop the arms but improve the pectoral (chest) muscles that hold up the breasts. While it is not likely that exercise will increase the size of a woman's breasts, the toning and strengthening of the pectoral muscles that support the breasts can make them appear more shapely.

THE EXERCISE
ARM LIFTS

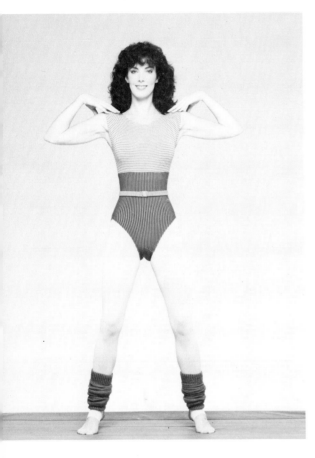
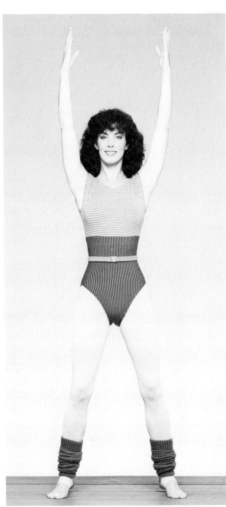

1 Start with hands on top of shoulders and elbows out to the side.

2 Reach hands as far as possible toward the ceiling with a feeling of tightening.

3 Return to shoulders.

4 Repeat eight times.

BENEFITS:	Improves posture, increases upper body strength. Muscles involved: Deltoids.
POSTURE:	Hold upper body erect with knees and shoulders relaxed. In all the arm exercises it is very important to keep the shoulders from lifting upward and to keep the chin in.
CAUTION:	Do not permit shoulders to lift. Keep ears in a direct line over shoulders. Keep chin in.

THE EXERCISE
SIDE ARM LIFTS

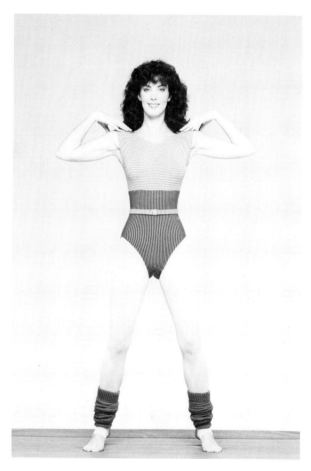
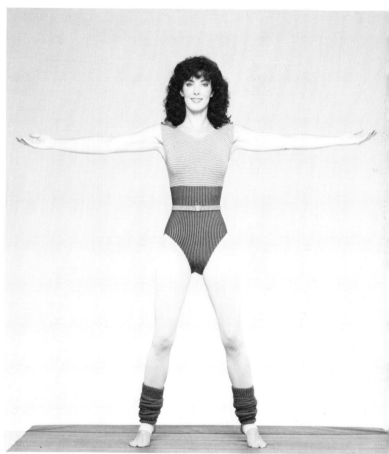

1 Start with hands on top of shoulders.

2 Unfold arms directly to the side with palms up.

3 Repeat eight times.

BENEFITS:	Increases arm and shoulder strength. Muscles involved: Deltoids, biceps and triceps.
POSTURE:	Keep elbows at shoulder level.
CAUTION:	Do not *snap* the elbow straight.

111 | UPPER BACK, ARMS AND CHEST

ARM CIRCLES

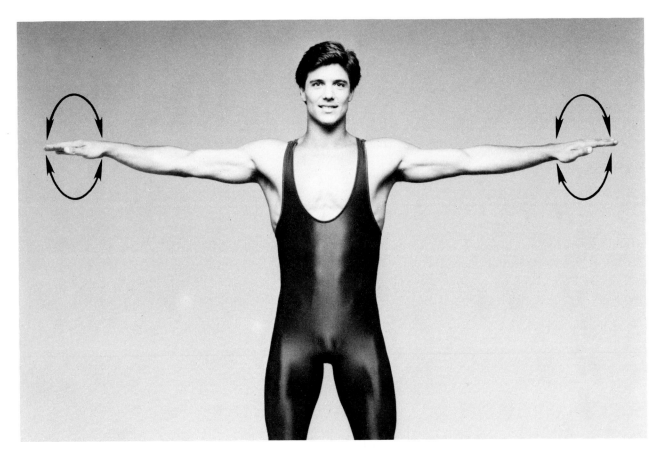

1 With arms still extended and palms down, move arms forward in small, tight circles.

2 Do one set of eight, two circles per count.

3 Reverse direction for another set of eight.

4 Repeat the exercise in both directions.

BENEFITS:	Improves arms and shoulder strength. Muscles involved: Deltoids and rotator cuff.
POSTURE:	Stretch arms as far as possible and keep them straight. Keep chin in.
CAUTION:	Do not lift shoulders upward. Keep chin pressed in toward chest.

LARGE ARM CIRCLES

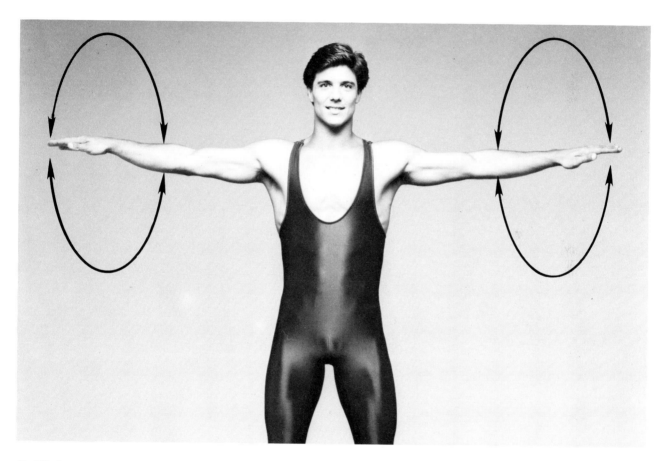

1 With arms extended to the side, flex palms.

2 Move arms in larger circles (one circle per count).

3 Do eight forward.

4 Reverse for eight.

BENEFITS: Improves arms and shoulder strength.
Muscles involved: Deltoids and rotator cuff.

THE EXERCISE
DOORKNOBS

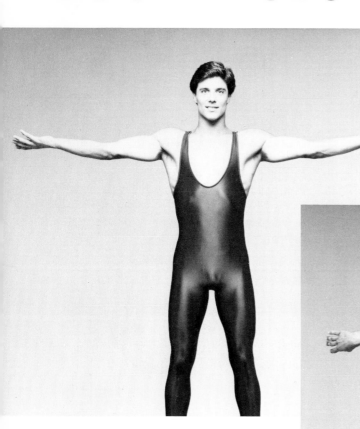

1 With arms extended to the side, and hands open and turned as if grasping large doorknobs . . .

2 . . . rotate arms as if opening a door to full range of motion.

3 Return to starting position.

4 Do four sets of eight in each direction.

BENEFITS: Improves shoulder strength and tones arms in general.
Muscles involved: Deltoids and rotator cuff.

POSTURE: Go to maximum rotation range.
Keep chin pressed in.

THE EXERCISE
BREASTSTROKE

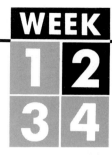

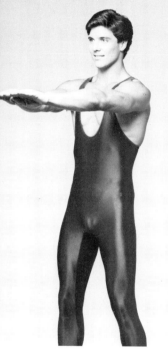

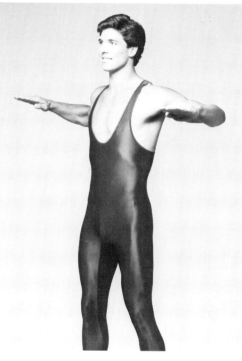

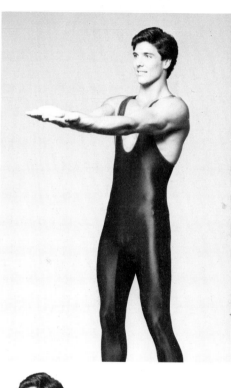

1 Extend arms forward, palms down, directly in front of chest.

2 Pull elbows back behind body.

3 Return to starting position.

4 Turn palms over and with arms straight, open arms to the side, extending as far as possible.

5 Return to beginning position.

6 Repeat two sets of eight.

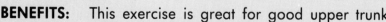

BENEFITS:	This exercise is great for good upper trunk posture. It stretches and strengthens the pectoral and upper back muscles. Muscles involved: Rhomboids and trapezius.
POSTURE:	Keep the hip stable, back straight, chest lifted.
CAUTION:	Do not allow the back to arch or release.

THE EXERCISE
PRESS
BACK

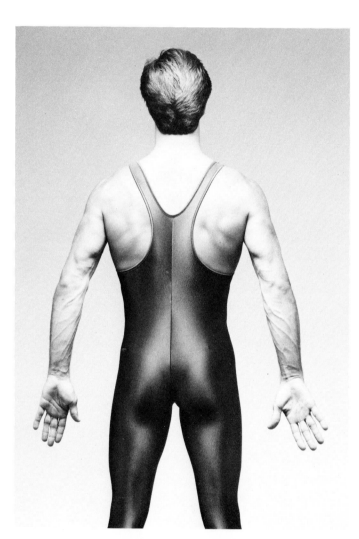

1 Arms are extended to the side in a seven o'clock position, palms facing back.

2 With small, firm, quick motions, press back.

3 Do four sets of eight.

BENEFITS: Good tension-releasing exercise. This exercise facilitates good posture, stretching the pectorals and strengthening upper back muscles.
Muscles involved: Rhomboids and middle trapezius.

CAUTION: Keep the body still, knees slightly bent. Keep chin pressed in.

THE EXERCISE
SIGNAL FLAG

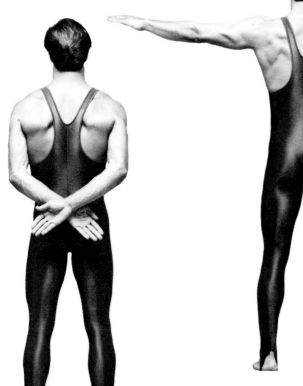

2 Open arms directly to side.

3 Bring arms over head and clap.

4 Bring arms back to side.

5 Return to cross-wrist position.

6 Repeat eight times.

7 End with arms overhead.

1 With arms still in seven o'clock position, cross wrists behind body.

BENEFITS: This exercise helps improve posture. Muscles involved: Trapezius, deltoids and rhomboid musculature.

POSTURE: Do not permit shoulders to fall forward. Keep chin pressed in.

CAUTION: Be sure to pause briefly in each position.

THE EXERCISE
LARGE DRUMBEAT

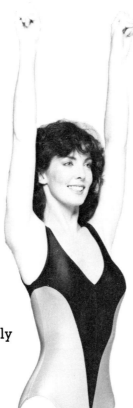

1 Begin with arms straight and directly overhead.

2 Clench fists.

3 Keeping arms straight, alternately lower them to chest level as if striking a drum.

4 Repeat for two sets of eight.

BENEFITS: Improves strength of large muscles of the trunk.
Muscles involved: Latissimus dorsi, pectorals, deltoids and trapezius.

CAUTION: Be sure to stop at chest level.

THE EXERCISE
SMALL DRUMBEAT

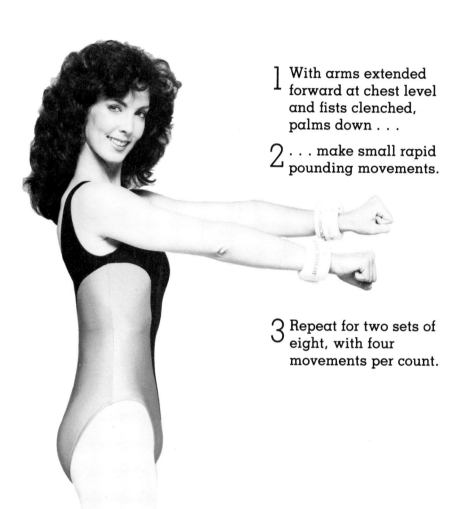

1 With arms extended forward at chest level and fists clenched, palms down . . .

2 . . . make small rapid pounding movements.

3 Repeat for two sets of eight, with four movements per count.

BENEFITS: Strengthens chest and shoulder muscles. Muscles involved: Deltoids, pectorals, trapezius and latissimus dorsi.

POSTURE: Keep arms tight.

CAUTION: Do not lean forward. Keep range of motion small. Keep chin in correct posture.

THE EXERCISE
CROSSES, PALMS UP

1 Extend arms forward with palms up.

2 Move right hand over left, crossing at elbows.

3 Alternate crossing left hand over right.

4 Do one set of eight at chest level.

5 Do one set of eight at hip level.

6 Do one set of eight at chest level.

7 Do one set of eight at eye level.

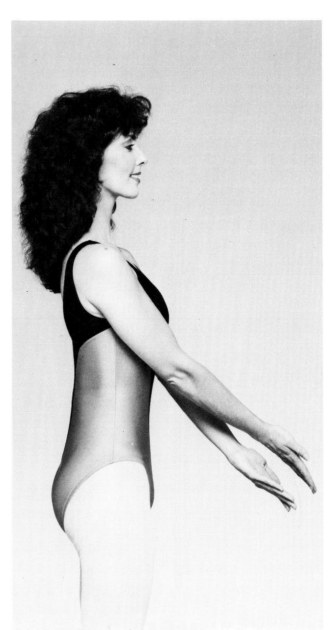
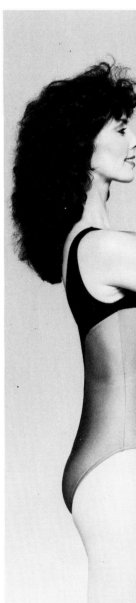

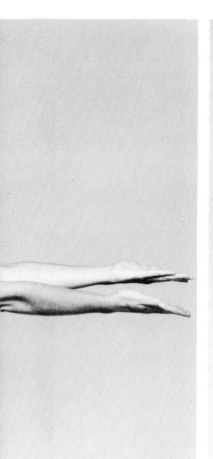

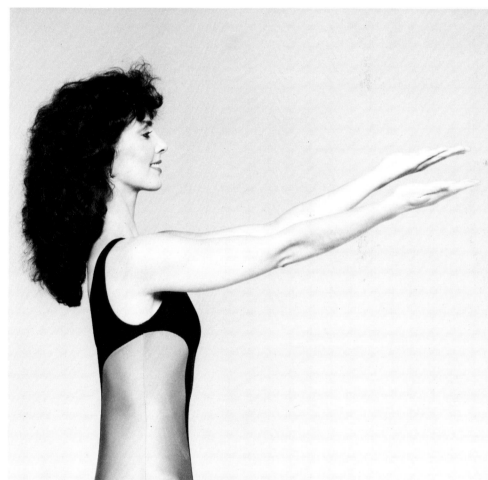

BENEFITS: Improves the tone and appearance of the muscles that support the breasts.
Muscles involved: Pectorals, deltoids.

CAUTION: Don't lean forward. Keep arms straight.
Keep chin pressed in.

THE EXERCISE
CLOCK

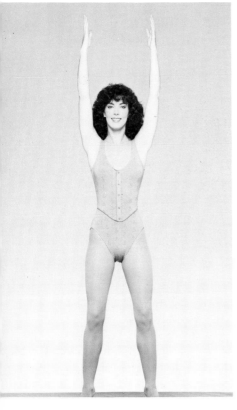

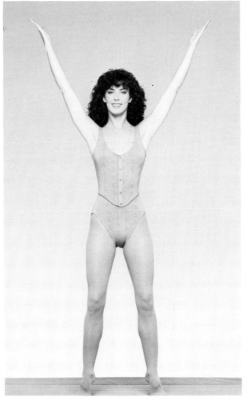

3 Repeat eight times.

4 Move arms to two o'clock and press back for eight counts with palms up.

1 Reach arms straight and directly overhead (twelve o'clock).

2 Press arms back in small and firm movements.

5 Move to three o'clock and press back for eight counts with palms forward.

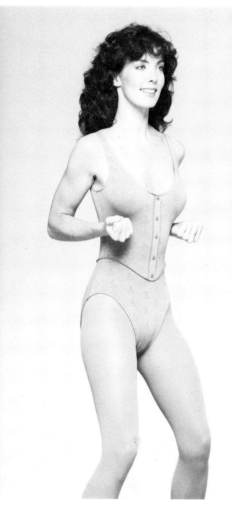

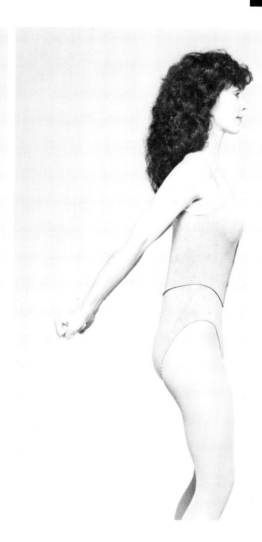

6 Lowering arms to four o'clock position and keeping arms behind body, make a fist, bend and extend arms for a count of eight.

7 Repeat entire series.

BENEFITS:	Improves muscles that hold chest up and shoulders back. Muscles involved: Upper back, triceps and deltoids.
CAUTION:	Do not permit back to arch.

THE EXERCISE
ANTIGRAVITY EXTENSIONS

1 With arms in four o'clock position, bend the upper body forward from the hips (keeping the knees bent and the back flat).

2 Continue to bend and extend arms keeping the elbows high.

3 Repeat for two sets of eight.

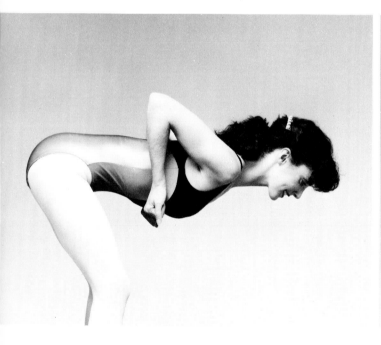

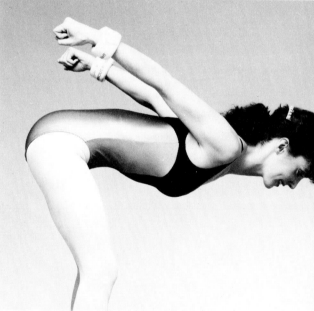

BENEFITS: Tones the upper arms and improves their appearance.
Muscles involved: Triceps and posterior deltoids.

POSTURE: Keep knees bent.
Keep elbows as high as possible.

CAUTION: Do not arch back and keep head and chest relationship as they are in standing.

THE EXERCISE
PEC PRESSES

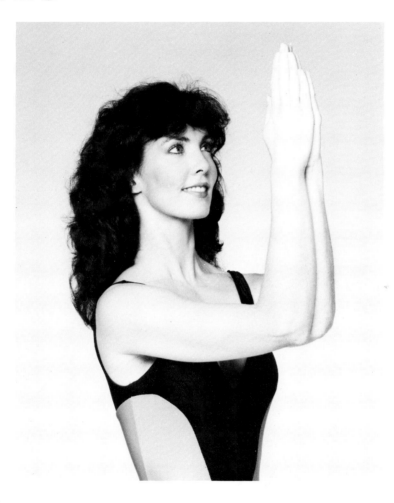

1 Bend arms and press palms together at forehead level.

2 Squeeze elbows together while tensing chest muscles.

3 Open elbows.

4 Repeat for four sets of eight.

BENEFITS: Improves the appearance of the chest. Strengthens the muscles that support the breasts.
Muscles involved: Pectorals, anterior deltoids.

CAUTION: Do not permit arms to drop.
Keep the stomach tight to keep back from arching.
Keep chin pressed in.

THE EXERCISE
PEC CROSSES

1 From Pec Press position, separate hands and alternately cross one elbow over the other.

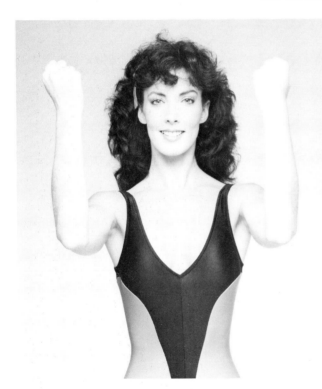 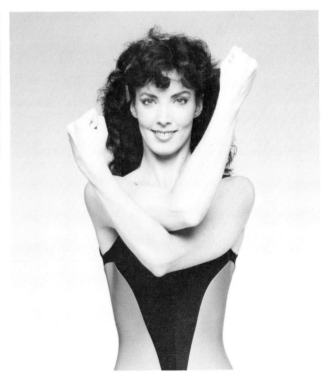

2 Repeat for two sets of eight.

BENEFITS:	Improves the appearance of the chest musculature. Improves breast support. Muscles involved: Pectorals, deltoids.
POSTURE:	Keep elbows high and bent at a 90-degree angle.

THE EXERCISE
PEC LIFTS

WEEK
1 **2**
3 **4**

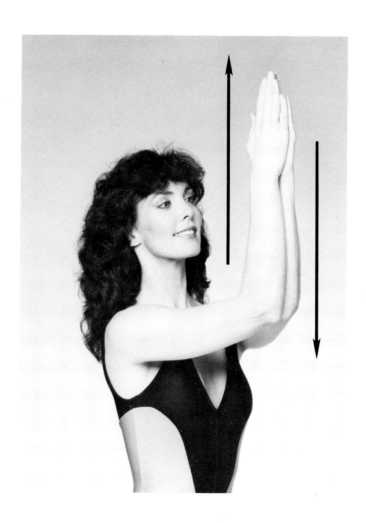

1 From Pec Cross position, bring hands and elbows together.

2 In this position, lift hands and arms directly toward ceiling.

3 Repeat for four sets of eight.

BENEFITS: Strengthens muscles of the chest and shoulders.
Muscles involved: Pectorals, deltoids and trapezius.

POSTURE: Keep chest lifted.

CAUTION: Do not permit elbows to drop or separate.
Do not allow chin to jut forward.

THE EXERCISE
TRICEP CLAPS

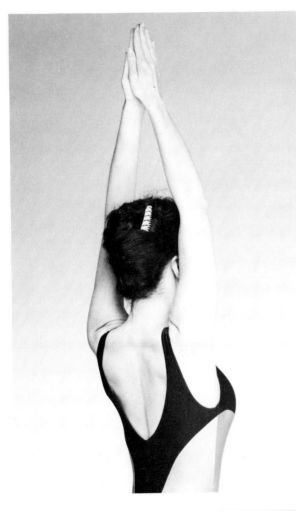

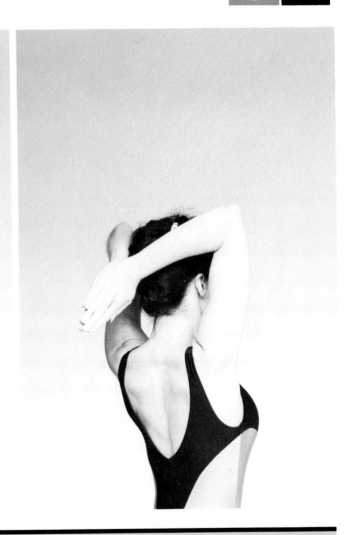

1 With arms overhead in line with ears, palms pressed together, drop hands behind head while keeping elbows high.

2 Drop and lift for two sets of eight.

BENEFITS:	Tones upper arms. Muscles involved: Triceps.
POSTURE:	Keep elbows close together. Do not arch the back.
CAUTION:	Do not permit head to drop forward. Keep stomach muscles tight.

THE WAIST

Everyone wants a trimmer waist.

This series of exercises starts to warm up the waist and back muscles and get them ready for the more strenuous abdominal series later in the program. Strong waist muscles not only give you that tapered look but help you to bend from side to side. This ability to bend makes exercising more vigorous and more beneficial.

As you do these exercises, become aware of the need to hold in the stomach muscles. Feel that posture improve.

Reshaping the waist is a two-part program. First, you must correct the poor nutritional habits that have overstuffed that stomach with the wrong foods—foods that bloated and added extra fat to the waist. Second, you must stretch the side muscles (external and internal obliques) to give shape and definition to the waistline. It is here that the extra padding (love handles, but who loves them?) can gather so very easily.

Now work on that waist.

REACH UP AND STRETCH DOWN

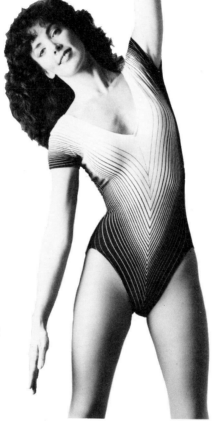

1 Stand with feet hip width apart.

2 With one arm extended straight toward the floor and the other arm extended toward the ceiling, bend sideways at the waist toward the floor.

3 Reach down for eight counts.

4 Change sides and repeat for eight counts.

5 Repeat in sets of four, two and one.

BENEFITS: Strengthens the side which you are bending toward and stretches the opposite.
Muscles involved: Obliques.

POSTURE: Keep hips stable, chest lifted, shoulders relaxed, knees slightly bent.
Do not lean forward. Keep movement small and concentrated.

CAUTION: Do not arch back.
Keep head and neck relaxed.

HAND-BEHIND-HEAD STRETCH

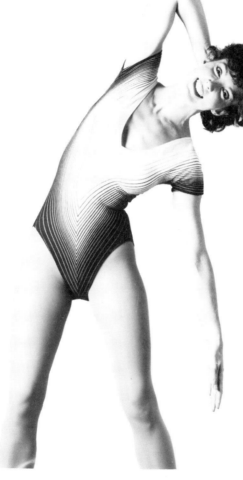

1 Stand with feet hip width apart, one arm down toward the floor. Bend top arm, placing hand on base of head.

2 Reach toward the floor with lower arm for a count of eight.

3 Repeat on other side.

4 Repeat in sets of four, two and one.

BENEFITS:	Tones and stretches the waist. Muscles involved: Latissimus dorsi and oblique abdominals.
POSTURE:	Keep shoulders directly in line with the hips as you bend. Keep the elbows out to the side, knees slightly bent.
CAUTION:	Do not arch the back.

THE EXERCISE

HALF TORSO TWIST

1 Stand erect with knees slightly bent.

2 With elbows open to the side, place hands on top of shoulders.

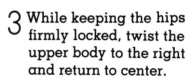

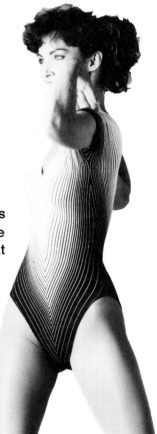

3 While keeping the hips firmly locked, twist the upper body to the right and return to center.

4 Twist for eight counts.

5 Repeat to the other side.

6 Continue in sets of four, two and one.

BENEFITS: Tones the waist.
Muscles involved: Internal and external oblique abdominal muscles.

POSTURE: Stand erect, abdominals tight and chin pressed in, knees slightly bent.

CAUTION: Do not permit hips or knees to move. Tighten buttock muscles.

COMPLETE TORSO TWIST

1 Stand erect with knees slightly bent.

2 With elbows open to the side, place hands on top of shoulders.

3 While keeping the hips firmly locked, do a complete twist from side to side at an increased tempo.

4 Do one set of eight.

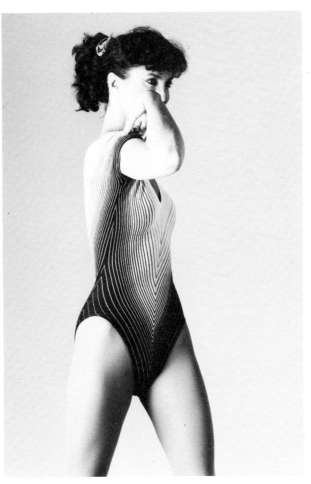

BENEFITS:	Tones waist and torso. Muscles involved: Oblique abdominals.
POSTURE:	Keep the hips still, in a controlled side-to-side motion. Keep erect posture, knees are slightly bent.
CAUTION:	Do not permit hips or knees to move.

THE EXERCISE
PUNCH TWIST

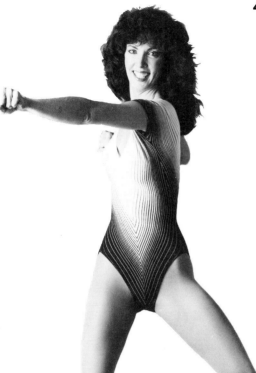

2 Do first set of eight with arms at chest level, second set of eight aiming toward the floor, and third set of eight at forehead level.

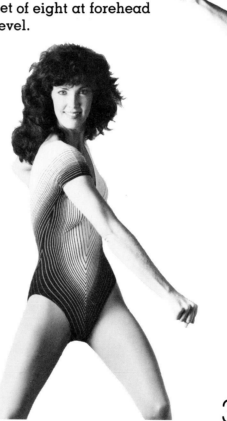

1 From the complete torso twist, begin to extend arms diagonally across the body in a punching motion.

3 Repeat entire exercise

BENEFITS:	Firms waist, chest muscles. Muscles involved: Pectorals, latissimus dorsi and internal and external obliques.
POSTURE:	Keep chin pressed in, stomach tight and knees bent more.
CAUTION:	Be sure to twist waist while punching.

THE EXERCISE
SCOOP PUNCH

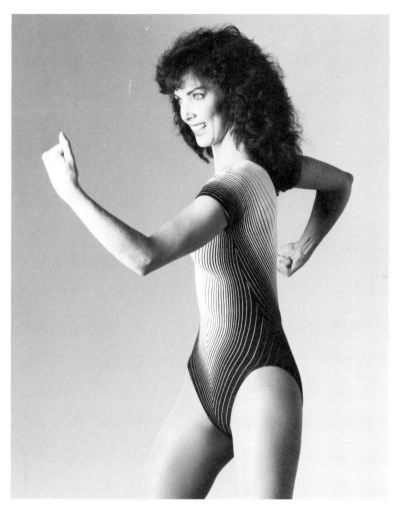

1 Starting from the position of the punch twist, hold arms (slightly curved) forward with palms up.

2 Alternately pull elbows back behind body while continuing the twisting motion in waist.

BENEFITS:	Works waist and arms. Muscles involved: Latissimus dorsi, pectorals, biceps and triceps.
POSTURE:	Keep chest lifted.
CAUTION:	Be sure to go to full range of motion. Keep knees bent and lower torso stable.

THE EXERCISE
PLIÉ STRETCH

1 Widen the stance so that the feet are more than hip width apart with toes pointed out to the side.

2 Hold arms straight out to the side.

3 While bending knees, cross arms in front of body.

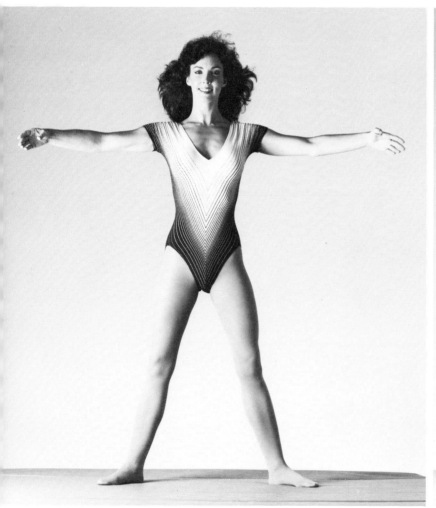

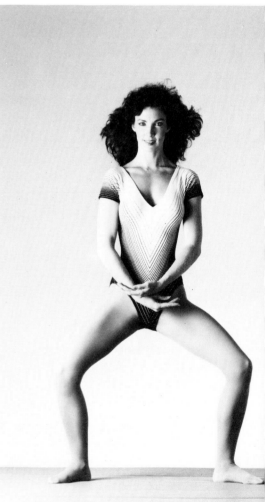

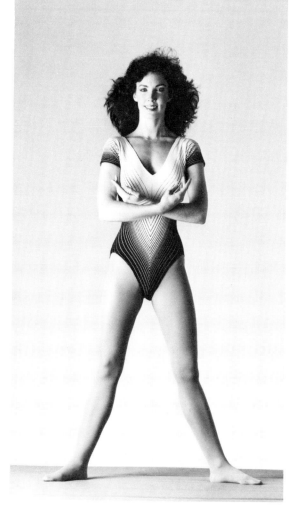

4 Straighten legs.

5 Bend knees, open arms and reach to the side with hands reaching up. Reach for two counts.

6 Repeat to the other side.

7 Do exercise four times.

BENEFITS:	Stretches waist to relax the muscles worked in this series. Muscles involved: Latissimus dorsi, quadriceps and obliques.
POSTURE:	Do not lean forward. Keep chin pressed, knees slightly bent.
CAUTION:	Do not lock the knees. Do not arch back. Relax the head.

THE EXERCISE
BUTTOCK ROCKING

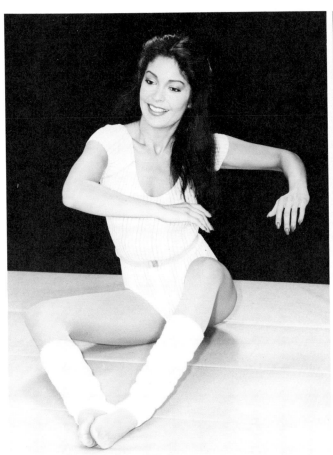
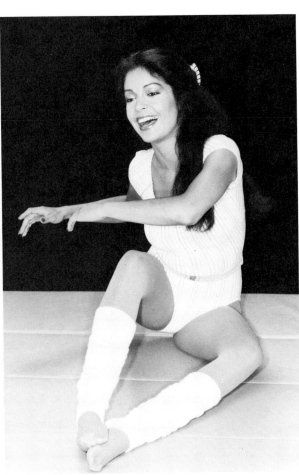

1. Sit on floor with legs bent and the soles of the feet together.

2. Rock from side to side twisting the body and lifting the knees.

3. Repeat for four sets of eight.

BENEFITS:	Maintains heart rate. Tones the waist. Strengthens the quadratus lumborum—an important back muscle. Muscles involved: Obliques and quadratus lumborum.
POSTURE:	Twist torso toward raised knee.
CAUTION:	Keep good, erect posture of upper trunk.

THE EXERCISE
BUTTOCK WALKING

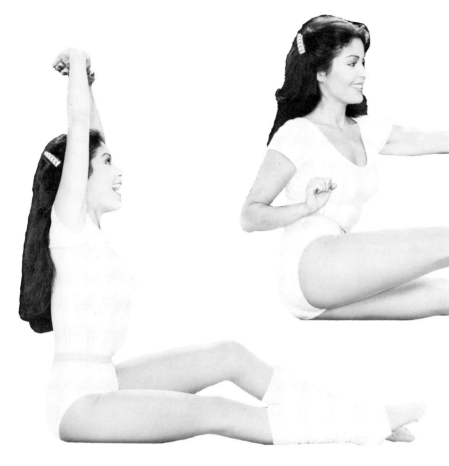

4 Alternately reach hands forward while hip-walking backward for eight counts.

5 Repeat exercise four times.

1 While sitting, extend legs directly in front of body.

2 Reach arms straight overhead.

3 Walk hips forward for eight counts.

BENEFITS:	Tones buttocks and waist. Increases heart rate. Muscles involved: Gluteus maximus and obliques.
POSTURE:	Keep upper torso erect.
CAUTION:	Do not arch the back. Keep chin pressed in and trunk held erect.

THE EXERCISE
BUTTOCK ROLLING

1 While sitting, extend legs directly in front of hips.

2 With hands on floor next to hips, bend and cross right knee over the left leg, touching the floor with the knee. Aim the heel toward the buttocks.

3 Repeat on other side.

4 Do two sets of eight.

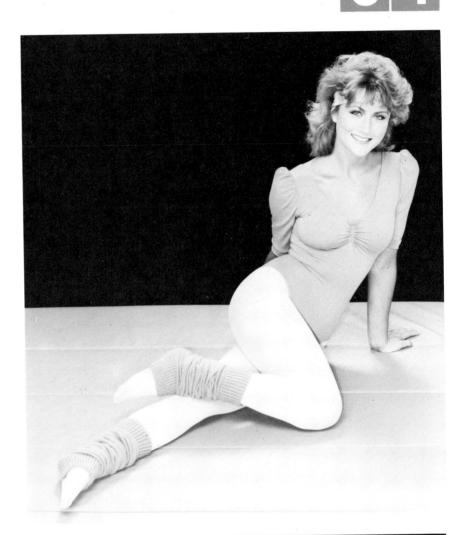

BENEFITS:	Trims waist and buttocks. Improves coordination. Muscles involved: Obliques and gluteus maximus.
POSTURE:	Keep trunk erect, chin pressed in.
CAUTION:	Do not permit upper body to lean back.

THE EXERCISE
BUTTOCK KICKING

1 While sitting with legs straight in front of body (hip width apart), swing the right leg (kept straight) across the left leg.

2 Return to starting position.

3 Alternate to other leg.

4 Repeat for four sets of eight.

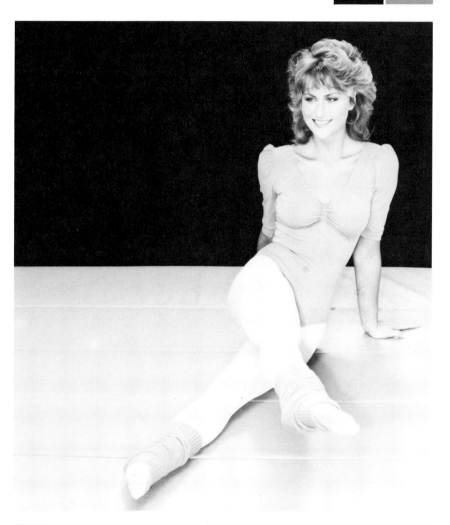

BENEFITS:	Works inner and outer thighs, buttocks. Muscles involved: Hip abductors and hip adductors.
POSTURE:	Keep trunk erect.
CAUTION:	Don't lean back.

ABDOMINAL SERIES

When you stand, do the stomach muscles sag and droop causing the whole body to have a dejected and haggard look? You need to strengthen the abdominal muscles.

Abdominal exercises are important because everyone wants to have a firm and tight tummy. But even more important than the visual attractiveness of the tight tummy is the development of strong abdominal muscles to support the back and buttocks. Tight stomach muscles also compress the internal organs into their proper positions so that they can function as efficiently as possible.

The abdominal muscles run from the base of the rib cage and attach to the pelvis. These muscles are vitally important to promote good posture. They not only keep the stomach from sagging but keep the pelvis backward and the back flat. This prevents the swayback.

Incidentally, the abdominal muscles are only responsible for the first 30 degrees of a sit-up. Once you lift higher, the hip flexor muscles take over. This means you should do the exercises exactly as directed and not try to push to a more exaggerated movement. If you substitute the hip muscles for the stomach muscles, you will run the risk of injuring the spine because the hip flexor muscles are attached to the front of the spine. Repetitive tugging on the spine will cause injury.

There are other important aspects of abdominal exercise that you should be aware of. One is that the back must always remain flat on the floor. If the abdominals are weak, and fatigue early in the series, the hip flexor muscle will substitute for the motion. As I have said, the hip flexors are attached to the lower spine and pull it forward into an arched back posture. This can be damaging to such a delicate structure as the back. If you are unable to keep the back flat during the entire series, you are doing too much for your current level of abdominal strength. If you have a backache after sit-ups, you are substituting the hip flexors for your weak abdominal muscles and you are in for far more serious trouble if you continue.

You should do as many sit-ups as you can without arching the back. If you arch up you should stop and rest 60 seconds and attempt just a few more. Then quit for the day. Tomorrow you will probably be able to do a few more in the correct form—with a flat back!!

Keep that back flat!

The neck is another area commonly injured in this series of the exercise program. There are two reasons: first, people have the misconception that the neck muscles will aid in the sit-up motion so they strain the head forward. This is untrue— these muscles are of no help whatsoever. So keep your head back and maintain the same relationship of your head to your shoulders as you would in standing. Second, people often allow their head to whip back and forth with the exercise movement. This uncontrolled movement is dangerous to the spine. The remedy is the same: keep the chin tucked in and maintain the head in one position—the correct position with your ears in line with your shoulders.

Think about that flat tummy you will have soon.

THE EXERCISE
ABDOMINAL CURL

1 Lie flat on floor with legs bent at the knees.

2 Place hands on top of thighs.

3 Slide the hands to the top of the knees, with upper body curling off the floor.

4 Repeat eight times.

5 On the last set, hold in elevated position for eight counts.

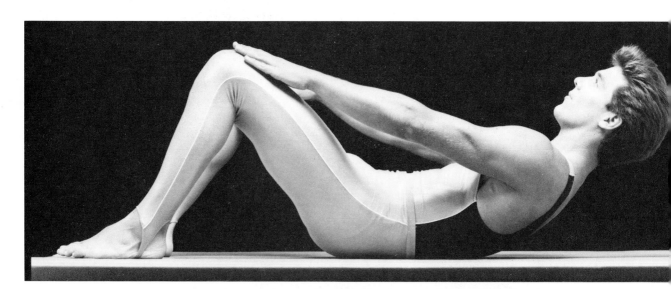

BENEFITS: Prepares body for abdominal series.
Warms up and tones abdominals.
Stretches back and shoulder muscles.
Muscles involved: Rectus abdominis and oblique abdominal muscles.

POSTURE: Press lower back into the floor. Keep chin tucked in. Ears are positioned in a direct line over shoulders.

CAUTION: Keep abdomen contracted, keep chin pressed in.

THE EXERCISE
ROPE CLIMB

1 Lie flat on floor with legs bent at the knees.

2 Reach toward ceiling, alternating arms as if climbing a rope. Clear shoulder blades.

3 Do three sets of eight.

4 Then clasp hands and hold with torso lifted for eight counts.

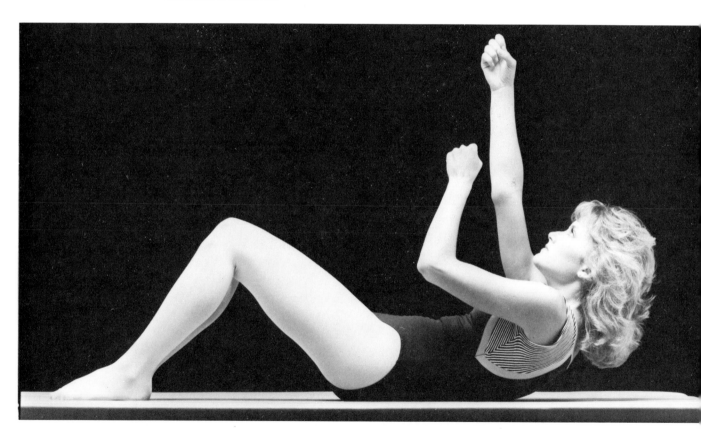

BENEFITS: Tones and strengthens abdominals. Muscles involved: Pectorals and rectus abdominis.

POSTURE: Keep lower back pressed into floor.

CAUTION: Do not permit back to arch. Keep abdomen contracted, chin pressed in.

THE EXERCISE

ONE LEG ROCK

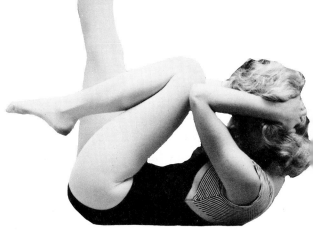

1 Lie on back, hands behind head, with one leg straight and extended toward the ceiling. Bend the other knee with the toe touching the floor.

2 Keeping the straight leg toward the ceiling, bring the bent leg toward chest, touch the knee with the elbows.

3 Return to starting position (toe pointed).

4 Do two sets of eight on the right leg and two sets of eight on the left.

BENEFITS:	Strengthens the abdominal muscles and hip flexor. Muscles involved: Rectus abdominis and hip flexor.
POSTURE:	Keep the lower abdominals pressed in.
CAUTION:	Be sure to keep the foot near the body as you lower it to the floor, and the knee bent.

THE EXERCISE
DOUBLE-TIME LIFTS

1 Lie flat with feet on floor (knees bent), with hand behind head (elbows open).

2 Lift upper torso toward ceiling clearing shoulder blades.

3 Do two lifts per count.

4 Repeat for two sets of eight.

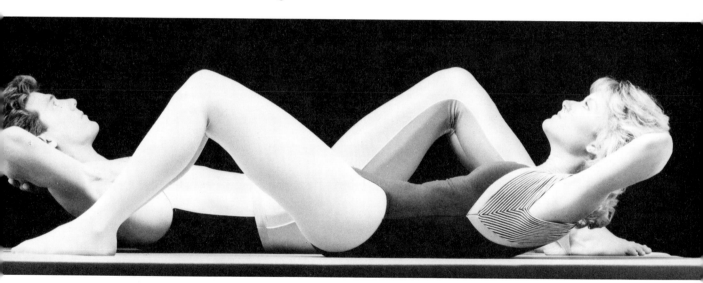

BENEFITS: Strengthens abdominals.
Muscles involved: Rectus abdominis.

POSTURE: Press in lower abdominals. Keep chin tucked in. Keep ears positioned over the shoulders.

CAUTION: This is not a big movement. Do not allow the back to arch up. Keep the abdominals contracted.
Don't strain the head forward.

THE EXERCISE
LEG-HIGH LIFTS

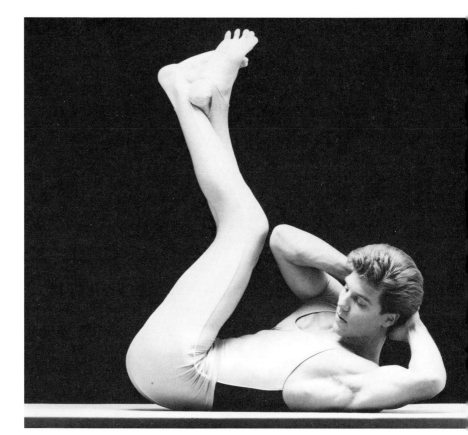

1 Lie on the floor with legs raised so that feet are higher than knees. Keep hips flexed greater than 90 degrees.

2 Cross ankles.

3 Interlock fingers behind head.

4 Keeping the small of your back on the floor, lift head and shoulders.

5 Twist the upper torso and try to touch left knee with right elbow.

6 Return to original position.

7 Repeat to other side (right knee to left elbow).

8 Do four sets of eight.

BENEFITS: Works the side abdominal muscles. Muscles involved: Internal and external obliques.

POSTURE: Lift upper torso as far as possible off floor.

CAUTION: Keep lower back on the floor. Keep hips flexed greater than 90 degrees.

90°

or: keep the thighs north of the straight up position.

THE EXERCISE
ALTERNATE LEG WALKS

1 Lie on the back with hands under buttocks.

2 Hold legs up with hips flexed greater than 90 degrees.

3 Lower one leg to the floor, but do not actually touch floor.

4 Lift other leg toward ceiling.

5 Alternate legs, giving each movement a full beat.

6 Repeat for two sets of eight on each leg.

BENEFITS:	Works the abdominals, front of the thighs and hip flexors. Muscles involved: Abdominals, hip flexors and quadriceps.
POSTURE:	Keep lower back pressed into floor.
CAUTION:	Keep lower back pressed into floor. Always keep one hip flexed greater than 90 degrees. This is achieved by keeping the thigh closer to you than it is to the floor.

THE EXERCISE

JAZZ LEG WALKS

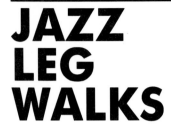

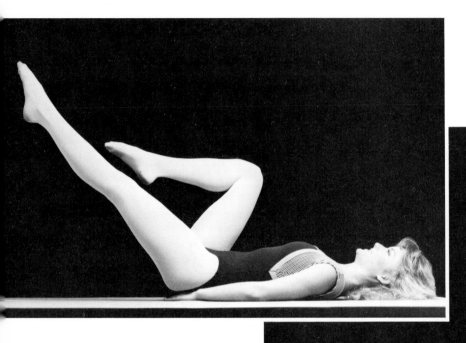

4 Repeat on other leg.

5 Do two sets of eight.

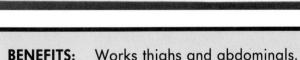

1 Lie on back with hands under buttocks.

2 Hold legs toward ceiling with hips flexed greater than 90 degrees.

3 While lowering left leg toward floor, bend the right leg, with right foot sliding along left leg with knee pulling toward chest.

BENEFITS: Works thighs and abdominals.
Muscles involved: Quadriceps and rectus abdominis.

POSTURE: Keep lower back pressed into floor.

CAUTION: Do not permit back to arch.
Keep hips flexed greater than 90 degrees.

THE EXERCISE
BICYCLE REACH

1 Lie on back with hands close to body, palms down.

2 Simultaneously bring one knee to chest while other leg extends forward in a bicycle motion, not to exceed a 90-degree angle.

3 Repeat on other side.

4 Do two sets of eight.

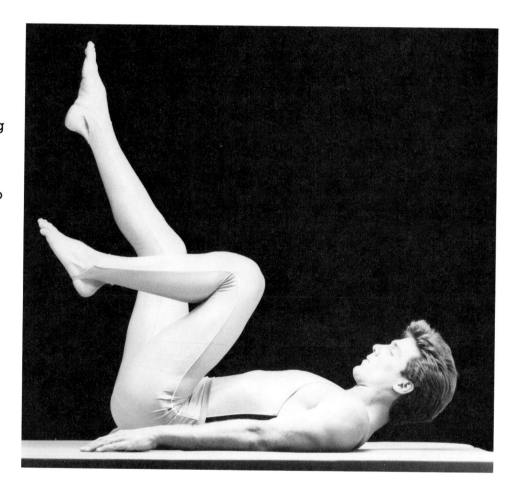

BENEFITS: Strengthens abdominal muscles.
Muscle involved: Rectus abdominis.

POSTURE: Keep lower back pressed into floor.

CAUTION: Do not allow the back to arch. Beginners should extend toward ceiling rather than straight out. As strength increases, aim the legs straight out.

THE EXERCISE
PELVIS STRETCH

1 Lie on back, knees bent, feet flat on floor.

2 Lift torso off the floor, pressing the pelvis toward ceiling.

3 Hold for four counts.

4 Repeat exercise.

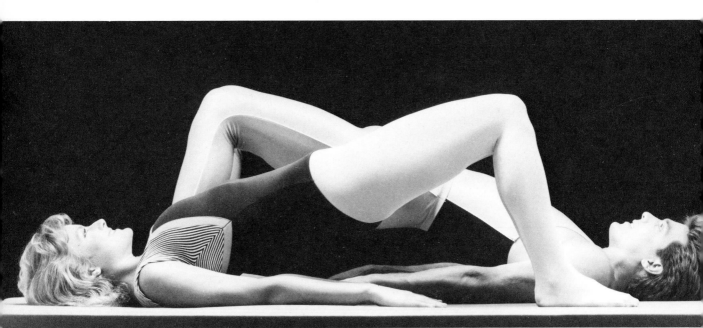

BENEFITS: To release and relax the abdominal muscles that have just been worked. To strengthen the back and buttock muscles.
Muscles involved: Gluteus maximus, hamstrings and lower-back muscles.

POSTURE: Keep shoulders and back relaxed.

CAUTION: Raise the pelvis only as high as your thigh. The torso and thigh should form a straight line.

THE EXERCISE
PELVIS LIFTS

WEEK
1 2
3 4

1 Lie on back, knees bent and hip width apart, feet flat on floor, arms extended with palms down.

2 While keeping the beltline on the floor, tilt pelvis and squeeze buttock muscles tightly; buttocks clear the floor.

3 Relax a little to prepare for the next squeeze, but do not release buttocks to floor completely.

4 Do eight lifts.

5 Hold in the raised position for eight.

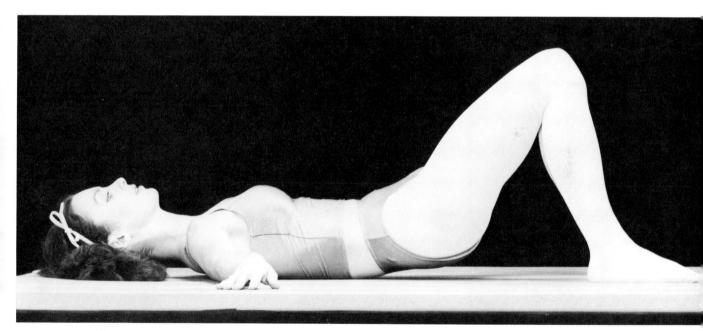

BENEFITS: Firms the buttocks.
Muscles involved: Gluteus maximus and minimus, hamstrings and lower-back muscles.

POSTURE: Keep back straight.

POSTURE: Relax upper torso.

CAUTION: Do not allow back to arch.
Keep the beltline on the floor, clear the buttocks only.

THE EXERCISE
PELVIC LIFTS, KNEES TOGETHER

1 Lie on back, legs bent, knees touching and feet hip width apart and flat on floor.

2 Lift the pelvis, keeping the back on the floor, and squeeze the buttock muscles. (The position of the legs helps to act as resistance to the movement for more benefit.)

3 Do eight lifts.

4 Hold for eight.

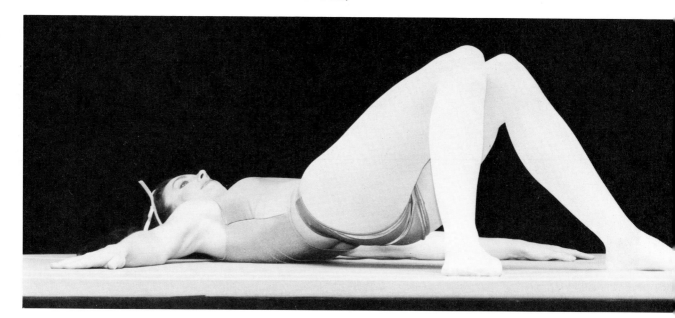

BENEFITS: Firms the buttocks and inner thighs.
Muscles involved: Adductor, gluteus maximus and hamstrings.

POSTURE: Keep back straight.

CAUTION: Do not allow back to arch.
Keep abdomen in.

THE EXERCISE
PELVIC LIFTS, FEET AND KNEES TOGETHER

1 Lie on the back, knees bent, feet flat on floor, knees and feet together.

2 While keeping the upper back on the floor, lift the pelvis and tighten the buttock muscles.

3 Do eight lifts.

4 Hold for eight counts with buttocks lifted.

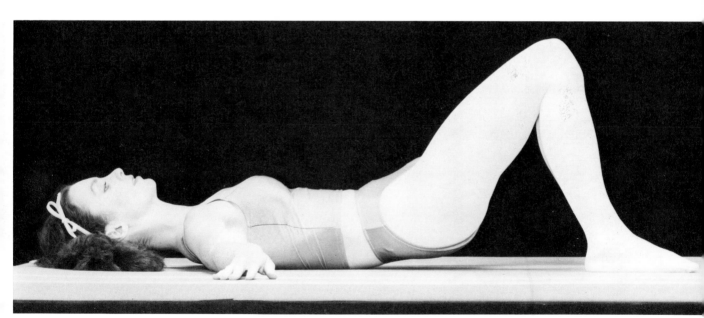

BENEFITS:	Works the buttocks and inner thigh. Muscles involved: Gluteus and adductor.
POSTURE:	Keep legs pressed firmly together.
CAUTION:	Do not allow the back to arch. Keep abdomen contracted.

PELVIC LIFTS, FOOT CROSSED TO KNEE

1 Lie on back, right leg is bent and the foot is flat on floor. The left foot is crossed over knee.

2 Lift pelvis and hips to ceiling while contracting buttocks. Keep the back on the floor.

3 Lift eight times.

4 Hold for eight counts.

5 Repeat to other side.

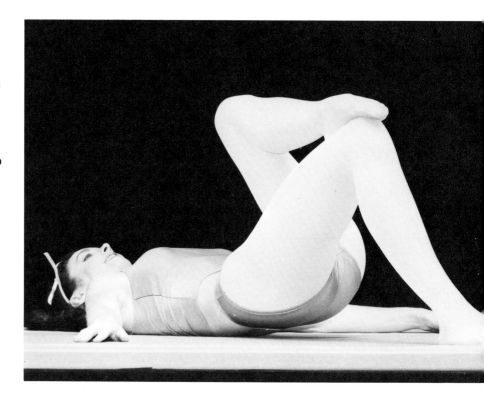

BENEFITS: Works buttocks, hips and thighs, isolating one leg.
Muscles involved: Buttock musculature.

CAUTION: Do not arch back.

BACK RELEASES

Watch that back!

I do not intend for anyone to follow the Body Design by Gilda program and come out of all this exercise with an injured back. Hurting the back is one of the major reasons why many people stop exercising. Because of this, I have made the back releases an important part of my program.

Do the back releases to keep everything aligned properly. These exercises are especially important at this point because you have just completed all those demanding sit-up movements of the abdominal series. The back muscles will be tight. These movements are designed to again relax and ease the pressures on the entire body. This is a strenuous and demanding (you are well aware of that fact by now) hour of exercising. It is extremely important to stretch and relax those taxed muscles.

This is a time to let that stress flow out of the body. Let up. Release that tension. Feel the improvement in that body already.

These back releases should become an important part of your *daily* life.

Back releases are those exercises illustrated here that have great importance in maximizing the benefits of the program while protecting the participant against injury. It is important to remember that injuries are felt after exercise sessions due to the natural tightening of muscles after they have been worked. Although damage may occur during exercise, it is most often felt after the body has cooled down. The reason being that the muscles tighten after cooling and the next move produces pain. Stretching the muscles after working (strengthening) them allows them to recover much quicker by returning them to their normal resting length.

Second, stretching muscles after a workout prevents the situation where tight and tired muscles may alter normal body mechanics and therefore place more stress on the joints of the body. This is particularly important when considering the back. The spine is made up of many joints and the movement of these joints under the strain of tight muscles can be damaging. The back releases are specifically placed in the program to stretch the muscles of the hips, buttocks and back after the abdominal series of exercises. The back muscles tend to tighten from abdominal work, so to improve recovery and protect the joints of the hips and spine, we have devised stretching exercises to release the tension from the hamstrings, buttocks and low-back musculature.

Do not skip any of these exercises, and remember the principle of stretching. Stretch to a discomfort, not a pain. The tension in the muscle should subside, not increase as you hold the stretch, and you must consciously relax the target muscles of each stretch to get the full benefit. Don't bounce.

ONE KNEE TO CHEST

1 Lie on back.

2 With your hands, pull knee toward the chest.

3 Hold for four counts.

4 Lower leg to floor.

5 Repeat with other leg.

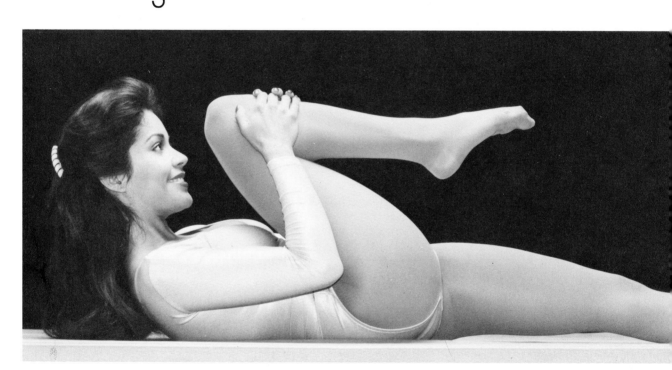

BENEFITS:	Stretches buttocks, lower back, backs of legs (hamstrings) and calves. Allows the back and pelvis to move more freely after class. Muscles involved: Gluteus, hamstring and gastrocnemius.
POSTURE:	Keep the leg on the floor straight.
CAUTION:	Keep lower back on floor. Do not pull the leg to the point of a painful stretch.

THE EXERCISE
KNEES TO CHEST

WEEK
1 2
3 4

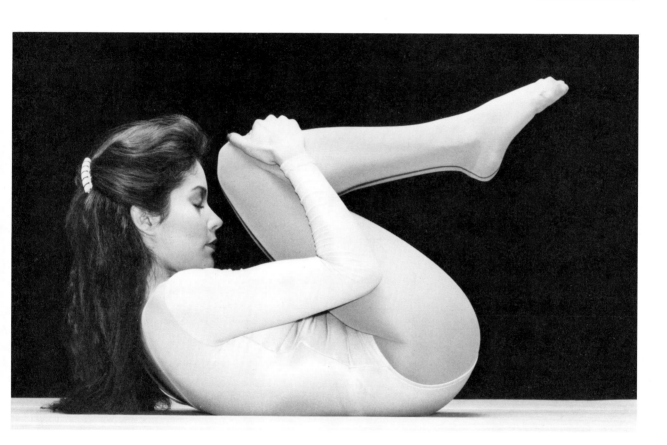

1 Lie down on your back.

2 Bend legs, bringing knees to chest.

3 Wrap arms around knees.

4 Press knees into chest and hold for a count of eight. Relax and feel the stretch.

5 Release slightly and repeat three times.

BENEFITS:	Stretches and relaxes the buttock and back muscles that have become tight from the work they have performed in the previous exercises. Muscles involved: Gluteus maximus, upper hamstrings and low-back muscles.
MORE BENEFIT:	Lift head toward the knees to stretch middle and upper back as well as the neck muscles.

THE EXERCISE
CROSS-OVER KNEE RELEASE

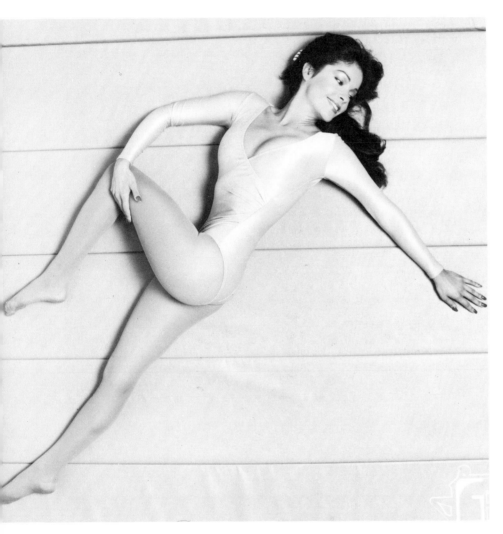

1 Lie on back with the right leg straight and the left leg bent toward chest.

2 Cross left leg over right.

3 Place right hand on left thigh; press leg toward floor.

4 Hold for a count of eight.

5 Return to first position.

6 Cross right leg over left and repeat exercise.

BENEFITS:	Allows free movement by releasing back tension.
	Muscles involved: Gluteus maximus and medius.
CAUTION:	Keep body relaxed.
	Palm and shoulders should stay on the floor.

THE EXERCISE
CROSS-OVER KNEE-DROP

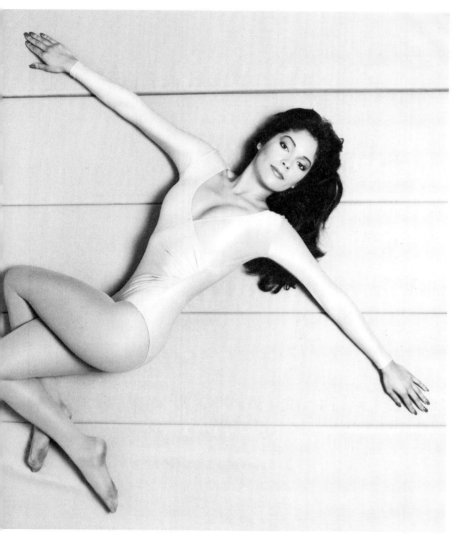

1 Lie on back with arms extended out to the sides, hands flat.

2 Cross left leg over right, both legs bent, and gently drop both legs to right side. Hold for a count of eight.

3 Return to center.

4 Cross right leg over left, and gently drop both legs to the left side. Hold for a count of eight.

BENEFITS: Allows free movement by releasing back tension. Muscles involved: Gluteus maximus and minimus.

CAUTION: Keep body relaxed.
Palms and shoulders should stay on the floor.

THE EXERCISE
YOGA RELEASE

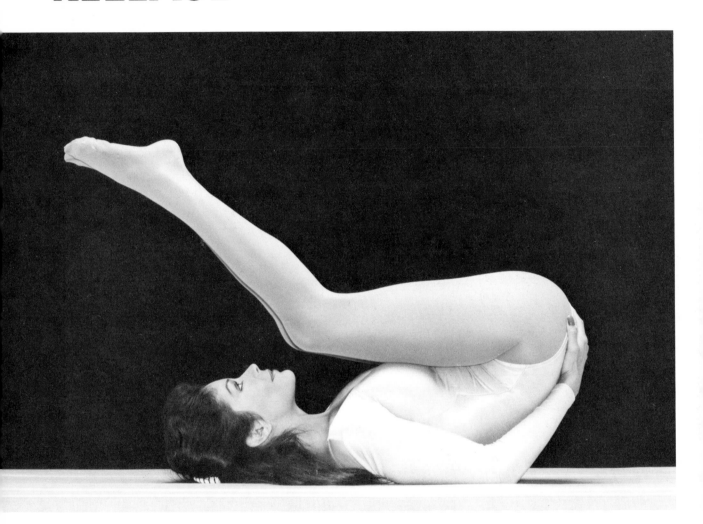

1 Lie on back.

2 Bring knees toward chest.

3 Roll back, bringing knees toward shoulders and feet behind head.

4 Hold for eight counts.

5 Bend knees for two counts.

6 Straighten for two counts.

7 Repeat exercise.

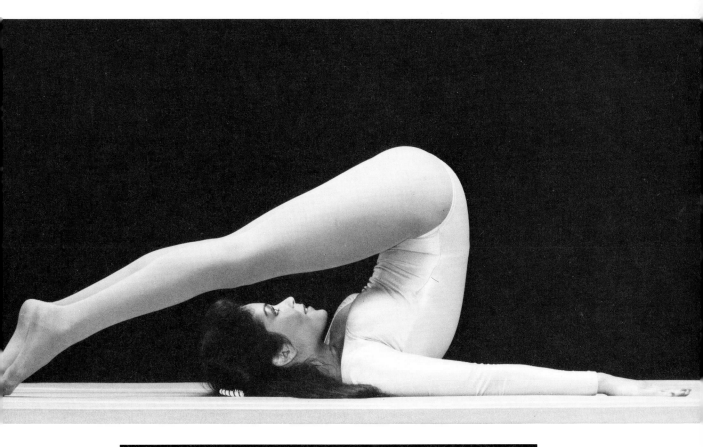

BENEFITS: Improves recovery and allows free movement. Muscles involved: Back, buttocks and hamstrings.

CAUTION: If you do not have the flexibility to bring the feet to the floor behind the head, then bring the knees to the shoulders. Be sure to keep head and neck facing ceiling. Do not turn your head to look to the side.

Pressure on/Pressure off

The importance of passive spine extension in any exercise program is that it offsets a life-style that usually finds our spines flexed. The rounding of the lower back is a common posture found. Not all chairs support us properly (with the spine slightly arched). Sofas and all soft seats cause the buttocks to sink forward and cause the lower back to round. Activities such as vacuuming, making beds, filing and lifting add to the amount of our day we spend bending forward.

What's the difference, you might ask?

Well, the spine is made up partly by cartilage discs that have a center portion of more or less syrup-like fluid that reacts to the pressures put on it. When the spine bends forward the disc is compressed in the front, forcing the fluid toward the back of the disc. This alters the normal biomechanics and is believed to cause more serious problems of the back such as ruptured disc (slipped disc) or nerve compression (pinched nerve). To offset the dangerous effects of flexion on the spine, passive back extension should be practiced regularly.

The exercise we present is a passive backward extension of the spine. This is achieved by a pressing up of the body using the arms. The back muscles remain relaxed, and the passive movement of the spine which is created occurs easily without excessive compression of the spinal joints. The compression that *is* created is localized in the back of the disc and is believed to recenter the fluids within the disc.

For many years doctors believed that back extension (backward movement) was dangerous and damaging to the back, probably for two reasons, the first being that many people with active back pain experience increased pain if they attempt to bend backward. This is because oftentimes when the disc is injured the spine falls out of straight alignment. Attempting to bend backward when the back is crooked or "shifted," as it is called in medical terms, may cause jamming of the spinal joints resulting in pain.

The second reason back extension exercises have received a bad name is because if done actively, that is if the back extension is achieved by an active contraction of the back muscles, there tends to be compression of the spinal joints that glide over one another. This can cause pain if the joint surfaces are roughened, as they are in many people.

In the last five years, the use of extension exercises has greatly benefited the conservative (nonsurgical) approach to disc disease. Physical therapists have learned to realign the vertebrae when they shift due to disc failure and perform passive extension exercises to recenter the inner disc fluid. The relief of the pressure that the bulging disc places on nerves and other pain-sensitive structures relieves the pain caused by this type of back injury. Passive back extension exercises done to a pressure on/pressure off sequence will keep the disc healthy and improve the way the spine moves during exercise and all activities of daily living.

THE EXERCISE
PRESSURE ON/ PRESSURE OFF

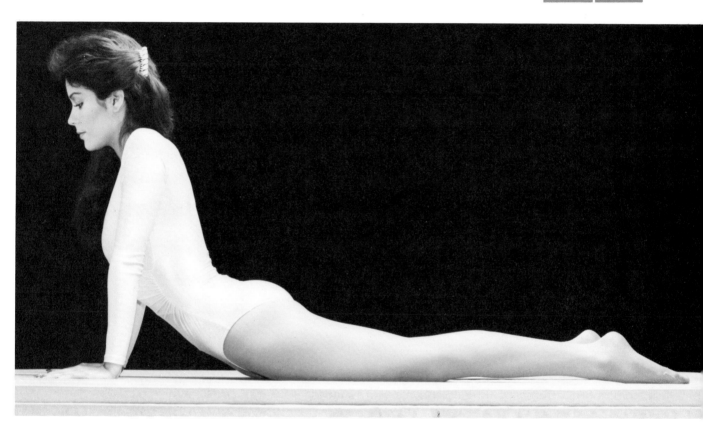

1 Lie face down on the floor.

2 Bend arms and place hands on the floor under shoulders.

3 Turn legs in so toes point toward each other.

4 Using arm strength only, straighten the arms. Do not stay in up extended position.

5 Bend arms to return body to original position.

6 Repeat five times.

BENEFITS:	Releases tension in the lower back caused by forward bending (flexing). Balances the pressure in the fluid of the discs. Muscles involved: Lower back muscles.
POSTURE:	Keep buttocks and back completely relaxed.
CAUTION:	Attempt to keep pelvis *on the floor.* *Keep buttocks relaxed.*

MAT STRETCHING

Stretching is the single most valuable aspect of physical fitness. It alone will offer the participant protection from injury, make all movements easier to perform, and correct poor posture which in turn can minimize all types of bodily malfunctions from joint and muscle problems to internal organ malfunctions.

The goal of stretching is to improve flexibility.

When muscles become tight from poor posture or from strengthening without stretching, the connective tissue will adapt to the shortened position. Connective tissue will shorten if left unstretched and is an "avoidable" result of aging. In fact, loss of flexibility is the one reversible aspect of aging and it is easily achieved. Simple stretching exercises done often enough (daily) will make even the tightest of muscles more flexible.

The principles of safe and effective stretching are easy but very important for the best results.

The first is the pain/discomfort principle, which states that you should never enter the painful range of a muscle stretch. The stretch can be progressed to the discomfort range but not become painful. The reason being that once pain is produced the muscle will respond by contracting to protect itself.

Second, is the subsiding tension principle, which states that the tension you experience with the stretch should subside as you hold the same position. If it increases you have overstretched and you should back off. If it decreases you can advance the stretch slightly.

In addition, all stretches should be held for 10 or more seconds, which allows the muscle to relax so you can stretch the connective tissue elements of the muscle.

Last, the positions of each stretch exercise should allow the body to relax into the stretch. If you have to exert any part of the body to maintain a position, the chance of your relaxing the target muscle is slim. This also requires that you know where each stretch should be experienced so you can relax the area entirely.

Stretching relieves tension, improves posture, hastens recovery after exercise and prevents injuries. It is the first thing I do in the morning and the last thing I do before bed, and it improves restful sleep.

THE EXERCISE
STRADDLE STRETCH

1 While seated on the floor, open the legs as far apart as comfortably possible.

2 Walk hands down one leg to ankle for four counts.

3 Hold for a count of eight. Feel the stretch in the inner thigh.

4 Walk hands up leg for four counts.

5 Repeat on the other side.

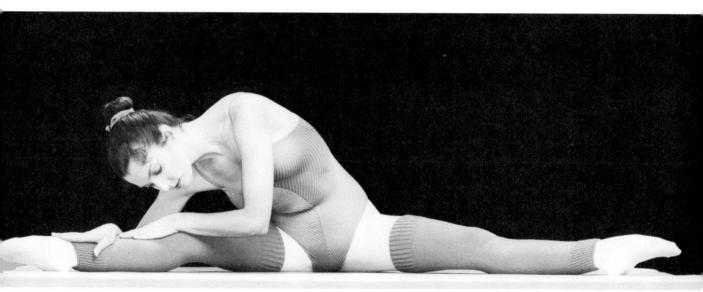

BENEFITS:	Improves biomechanics of leg, pelvis and back by stretching a typically tight set of muscles that anchor on the pelvis. Stretches inner thigh (adductor) and hamstring and back muscles. Muscles involved: Gracilis and hamstrings.
POSTURE:	Keep knees open and legs rotated out. *Keep both hips on the floor.*
CAUTION:	Do not force stretch. Do not enter the pain range of the stretch.

THE EXERCISE
BALLET STRADDLE

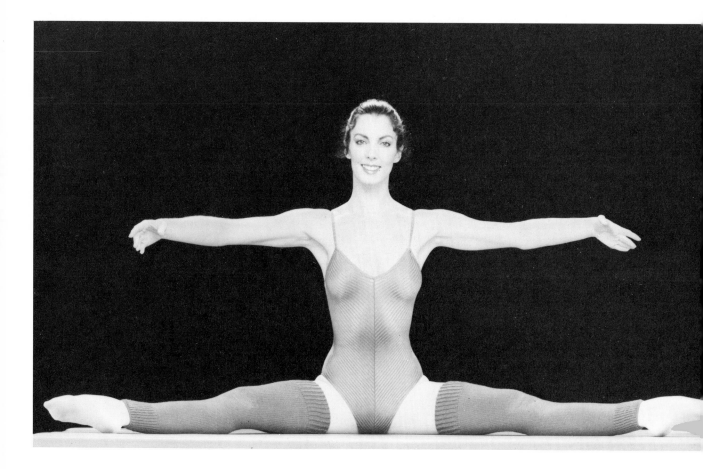

1 Sit on floor with legs apart.

2 Open arms to the sides at shoulder level.

3 Bend body to the left, reaching right arm overhead toward left ankle.

4 Hold for eight counts. Feel back and side stretch.

5 Repeat on other side.

6 Do twice on each side.

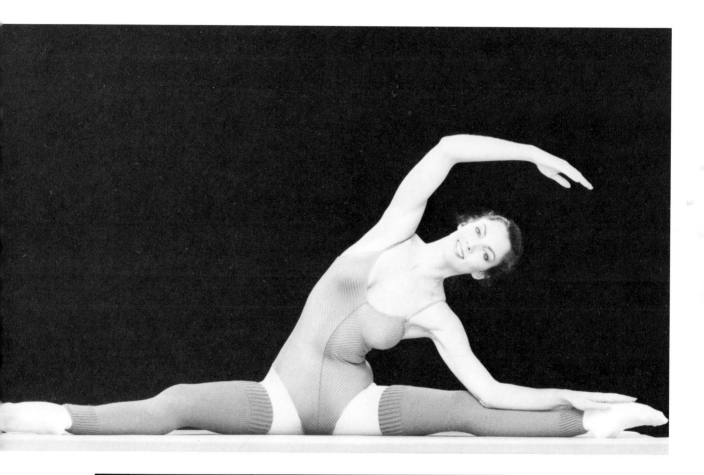

BENEFITS:	Improves movement and protects against spine injury by stretching typically tight muscles. Muscles involved: Inner thigh, obliques, lower back, latissimus dorsi and quadratus lumborum.
POSTURE:	Keep knees turned back. Keep raised arm and shoulder open. Do not turn toward knee.
CAUTION:	Do not force the stretch. Do not cause pain in the stretch.

REACH FOR TOES

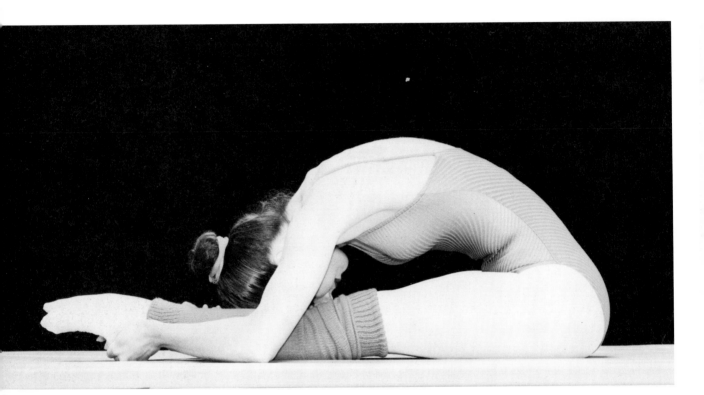

1 Sit on floor with legs straight in front of hips.

2 Walk hands down legs to toes in four counts.

3 Hold and relax for a count of eight.

4 Reach farther for a count of eight.

5 Walk up legs for a count of four.

6 Repeat exercise.

BENEFITS:	Prevents against back injury by returning the very important back muscles to their normal resting length. Muscles involved: Hamstrings.
POSTURE:	Do not bend legs.
CAUTION:	Do not force stretch. Do not enter the pain range of the stretch.

THE EXERCISE
SWIM STRETCH

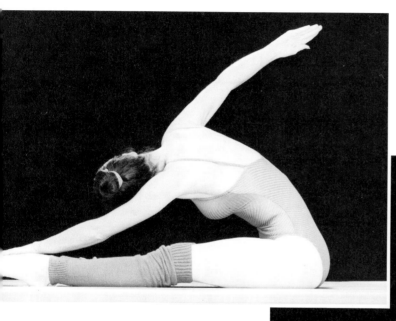

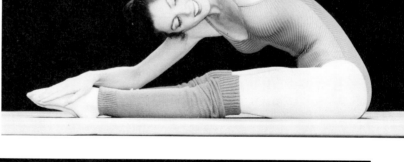

1 Sit on floor with legs straight in front of hips.

2 Reach the left hand toward the toes as the right hand circles behind and overhead in a swimming motion.

3 Repeat with right arm.

4 Do two sets of eight exercises.

BENEFITS:	Loosens the shoulders and upper back and begins to elevate the heart rate. Muscles involved: Hamstrings, buttock, back and shoulder muscles.
POSTURE:	Keep legs straight, and reach as far as possible.
CAUTION:	Relax the shoulders. Keep head relaxed and centered.

LEGS, HIPS AND THIGHS

Get ready to start developing great legs . . . a fabulous fanny . . . and firm thighs.

The following series of exercises, if done correctly, will not only resculpture those problem areas but will strengthen the body.

But be careful!

It is very important to do the side leg lift exercises correctly.

The goal of these exercises is to strengthen the muscles of the outer hip and upper thigh. These outer buttock and hip muscles are important in all walking and running activities and will pull the buttock flesh tighter and make the entire buttock and outer thigh area more toned and shapely.

So they are important, but if overdone, or done incorrectly, they can cause problems with the spine.

The major precaution in these exercises is to keep the pelvis *still*—that is to eliminate all rocking motion of the pelvis. The reason being that the spine and pelvis are obviously attached and rocking of the pelvis will cause acute side bending of the lower spine. This can be damaging. The safeguard against this excessive movement is to keep the side-lying leg lifted within the range of motion at the hip, which is approximately 45 degrees only. Any further upward movement of the leg will be taking place at the joints between the spine and the pelvis.

Lift the leg approximately 12 to 18 inches off the floor only. You must keep the toe and kneecap pointed forward. Do not turn out or let the leg go higher.

By elevating the upper torso and by limiting the range of motion of the leg lift we have safeguarded the spine and isolated the muscles *we truly wish* to exercise in this routine—the outer buttock and hip muscles (gluteus medius and minimus, the tensor fasciae latae and some of the gluteus maximus).

Other common but dangerous variations of this exercise include flexing the hip to a right angle in front of the body and pushing up higher toward the head. This will strain the hip flexor (iliopsoas) and will strain the back and spinal muscles.

The other commonly seen problem with these exercises is that they are often overdone. They should be done in sets of eight or ten with a brief rest in between sets to allow for the muscle to relax and allow *new blood to flow in* and old blood (full of waste products) to evacuate. If overdone, the muscle will spasm and cramp, causing pain and often long-term problems.

THE EXERCISE
SIDE LEG LIFTS

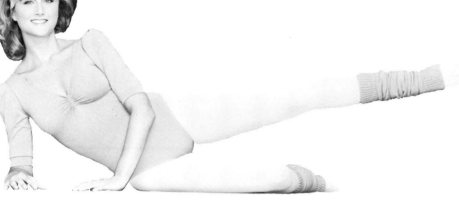

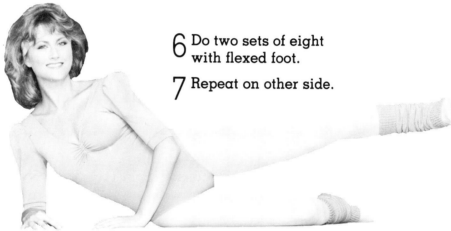

1 Lie on side with weight supported on elbow and hip, with side of torso lifted off floor as far as possible.

2 Bend bottom leg and place bottom knee forward.

3 Extend top leg in line with hip.

4 Press top hip forward in line with bottom hip.

5 Raise and lower leg for two sets of eight (keep toes pointed).

6 Do two sets of eight with flexed foot.

7 Repeat on other side.

BENEFITS:	Improves appearance of buttocks. Strengthens and tones outside of leg and hip. Muscles involved: Gluteus medius and minimus, tensor fasciae latae and gluteus maximus.
POSTURE:	Keep upper torso lifted as high as possible. Do not allow back to arch back.
CAUTION:	Do not permit pelvis to move during this exercise. Keep neck and shoulders relaxed. We have protected the spine by keeping the pelvis from rocking up and down with each lift. This is accomplished by propping the upper body on the elbow.

THE EXERCISE
CIRCLE LIFTS

WEEK

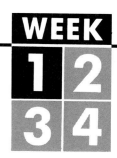

1 2
3 4

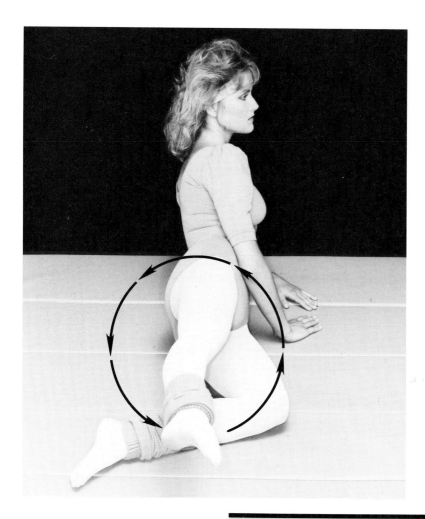

1 Lie on side with weight supported on elbow and hip, with side of torso lifted off floor as far as possible.

2 Bend bottom leg and place bottom knee forward.

3 Extend top leg in line with hip.

4 Press top hip forward in line with bottom hip.

5 With toe pointed, circle top leg forward for eight counts.

6 Reverse leg backward for eight counts.

7 Repeat in both directions.

8 Repeat exercise on other side.

BENEFITS:	Improves appearance of buttocks. Tones outer thigh and hip. Muscles involved: Gluteus medius, minimus, tensor fasciae latae and gluteus maximus.
POSTURE:	Do not allow low back to arch.
CAUTION:	Do not permit torso to move. Keep leg in safe range, at hip height.

THE EXERCISE
ACCORDION LIFTS

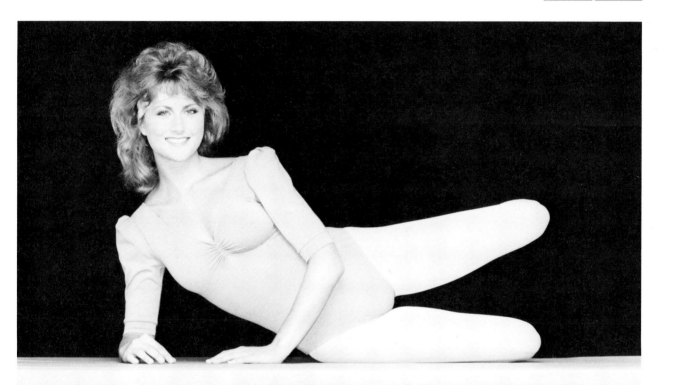

1 Lie on side with knees bent and pressed behind the line of the hips.

2 Lift the top leg, keeping the foot and knee in one horizontal line.

3 Lower the leg and press legs together.

4 Repeat for two sets of eight.

5 Repeat exercise on opposite side.

BENEFITS:	Strengthens and tones outside of leg, hips and buttocks. Muscles involved: Gluteus medius, minimus.
POSTURE:	Do not permit legs to go forward while lifting. Do not open the leg.
CAUTION:	Be sure to keep back in straight alignment.

THE EXERCISE
EXTENDED ACCORDION LIFT

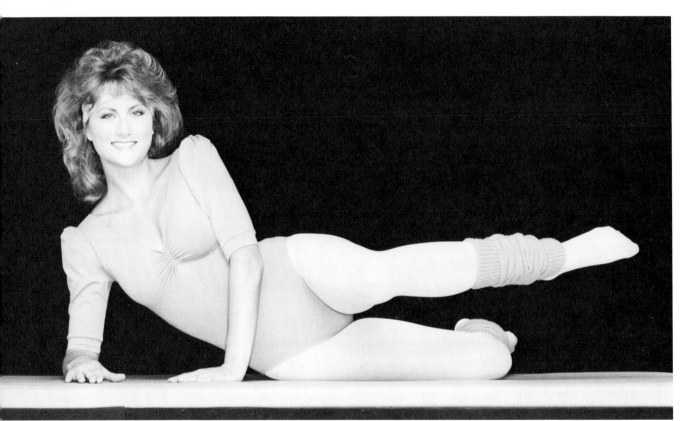

1 Lie on side, propped up on elbow.

2 Keep both knees bent at a 90-degree angle.

3 Lift top leg to a 45-degree angle and lower to touch bottom knee.

4 Repeat eight sets.

5 Repeat exercise on opposite side.

BENEFITS:	Works outer and inner thighs and buttocks. Muscles involved: Tensor fasciae latae, gracilis and gluteus medius and minimus.
POSTURE:	Keep leg in line with hips when extending the leg.
CAUTION:	Straighten the knee gently. Keep back in proper alignment.

THE EXERCISE
OUTER THIGH T-LIFT

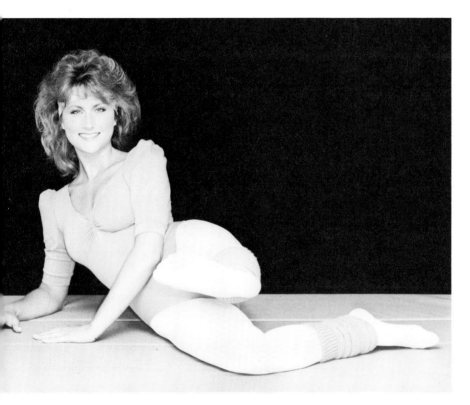

3 Flex hip so other leg is 45 degrees in front of body.

4 Lift and lower leg for a count of eight.

5 Do one set of eight.

6 Repeat on other side.

1 Lie on side with weight supported on elbow and hip, with side of torso lifted off floor as far as possible.

2 Bend bottom leg and place bottom knee forward.

BENEFITS:	Improves, strengthens and tones outer thighs and buttocks. Muscles involved: Tensor fasciae latae, gluteus medius and minimus.
POSTURE:	Keep upper body slightly forward.
CAUTION:	Do not permit hip to move. Keep back flat. Do not bring top leg forward more than 45 degrees from straight position.

THE EXERCISE
INSIDE THIGH LIFTS

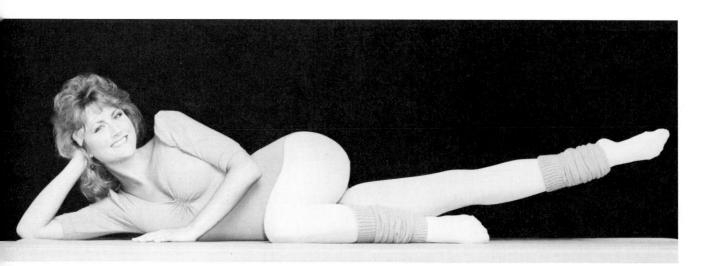

1 Lie on side resting on elbow.

2 Relax top leg down to floor.

3 Extend bottom leg straight in line with hip and body.

4 Lift lower leg up and down.

5 Repeat eight times.

6 Flex the foot.

7 Repeat eight times.

8 Repeat exercise with leg bent behind.

9 Repeat entire series on opposite side.

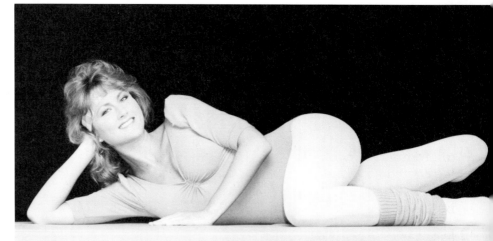

BENEFITS:	Tones and firms inner thighs. Muscles involved: Adductor group.
POSTURE:	Point knee and toes forward.
CAUTION:	Do not allow pelvis to drop back.

THE EXERCISE
FIRM BUTTOCKS LIFTS

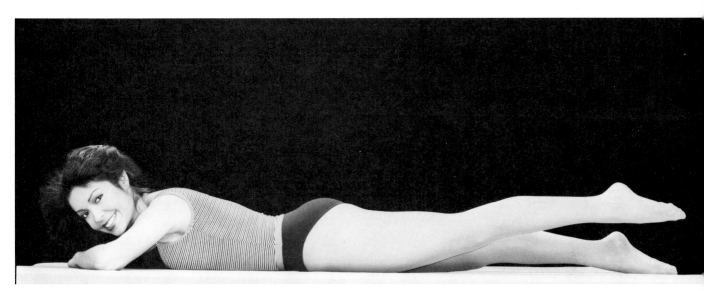

1 Lie flat on your stomach on the floor.

2 With legs straight, alternately lift each leg off the floor one at a time, tensing the buttocks.

3 Lift to a count of eight for each leg.

BENEFITS: Strengthens the important muscles for back stability. Improves the appearance of the buttocks and upper thighs.
Muscles involved: Low-back muscles, erector spinae, gluteus maximus and hamstrings.

POSTURE: Press pelvis into floor, keeping abdomen tight. Keep head in good alignment.

CAUTION: Do not lift legs higher than a few inches. Protect the spine by limiting the amount of leg raising to a few inches. This will keep the back arch within a safe range. Tightening the stomach prevents spine arching beyond its safe range. The arching of the back in this type of exercise is of the "active" type, which is stressful to the spinal joints.

THE EXERCISE
CROSS-ANKLE LIFTS

1 Lie face down, head on hands.

2 Cross ankles, keeping legs straight.

3 While tensing the buttocks, lift the legs off the floor approximately two inches.

4 Lower feet to floor.

5 Repeat eight times.

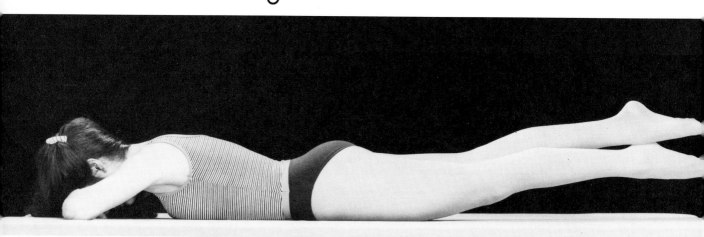

BENEFITS: Firms buttocks and thighs.
Muscles involved: Erector spinae, gluteus maximus and hamstrings.

POSTURE: Keep front of pelvis on the floor.

CAUTION: People with lower-back problems should keep thighs on floor. Keep abdominals tightened.
We have protected the spine by limiting the back arch to a small degree. This exercise strengthens the very important muscles in the low back without stressing the spinal joints.

THE EXERCISE
LEG LIFTS
DIRECTLY BEHIND

These exercises are usually done in the all-fours position or lying flat on the stomach, and are very important to strengthen the muscles of the back which stabilize the spine. They work the spine. They also work the buttock muscles and the upper thigh and have obvious aesthetic value. The problem is that they are commonly performed in excessive range of motion. Any backward movement of the upper leg that exceeds the range of motion possible in the hip joint itself will stress the joints of the lower spine by causing the pelvis to tilt.

The prime mover of any backward leg movement is the gluteus maximus muscle, which makes up the bulk of the buttock flesh.

If the exercises are performed in the proper range they will also work the back muscles, as they stabilize the spine and pelvis during movement of the leg. Excessive lifting of the thigh will cause damage to the spine that might not be painful now but can cause problems in the future.

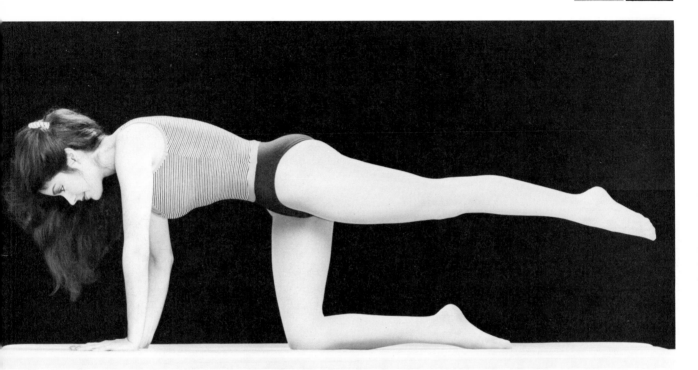

1 Begin on hands and knees.

2 Extend one leg straight behind body. Raise leg to hip level and lower.

3 Repeat eight times.

4 Do other side.

BENEFITS: Very important exercise to strengthen back muscles that move the spine.
Muscles involved: Low back, erector spinae, buttocks and upper hamstring.

POSTURE: Do not raise leg higher than hip height. Keep hips level.
Keep abdomen pulled in!!
Keep head in good alignment.

CAUTION: Do not allow back to arch! Do not allow pelvis to tilt either down or up.
We have protected the spine by eliminating back arching and keeping stomach tight.
We have isolated the movement to the hip joint only in order not to stress the joints of the back.

THE EXERCISE
KNEELING LEG CURLS

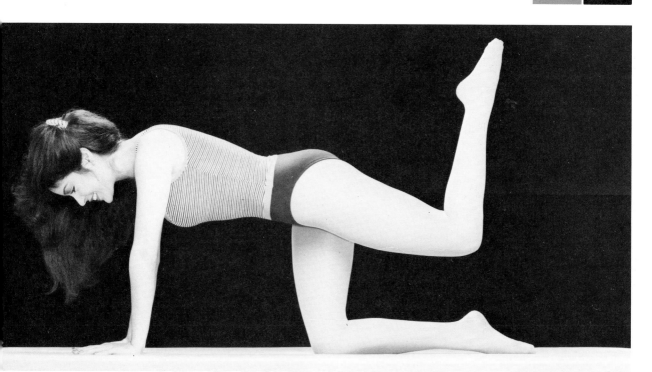

1 On hands and knees, bend and extend knee at hip level.

2 Do two sets of eight.

3 Repeat on other side.

BENEFITS: Strengthens the back, buttocks and upper thighs.
The buttocks and entire hamstrings are worked in this exercise.
Muscles involved: Erector spinae, gluteus maximus and hamstrings.

POSTURE: Keep thigh at hip level.
When the knee bends, keep head in straight posture—chin tucked in and ears aligned with shoulders.
Keep eyes focused on floor.

CAUTION: Protect back by eliminating arch of the back.
Keeping the abdominals tight will prevent arching of the back.

THE EXERCISE
CATBACK

1 In the all-fours position, with the hands directly below the shoulders and the knees directly below the hips . . .

2 . . . tighten the abdominal muscles to pull the lower pelvis forward. Round the back and shoulders like a cat's hunched back.

3 Relax the back as you tighten the stomach. Feel the stretch along the entire length of the back.

4 Repeat twice to an eight-count hold.

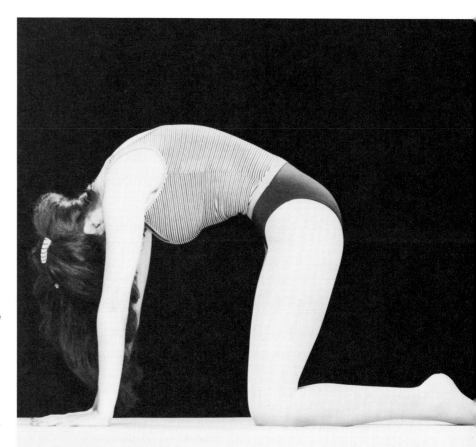

BENEFITS: Stretches the spinal muscles that cause swayback and that have tightened by the previous exercises performed.
Muscles involved: Erector spinae, rhomboids, middle trapezius, buttocks and abdominal musculature.

POSTURE: Keep head and neck relaxed by allowing the head to hang relaxed.

CAUTION: Keep the head relaxed and let it hang.

THE EXERCISE
PRAYER

1 In the all-four catback position, bend the elbows and move your buttocks back so your buttocks and heels touch.

2 Feel the stretch increase throughout the length of the back muscles.

3 Hold for one count of eight.

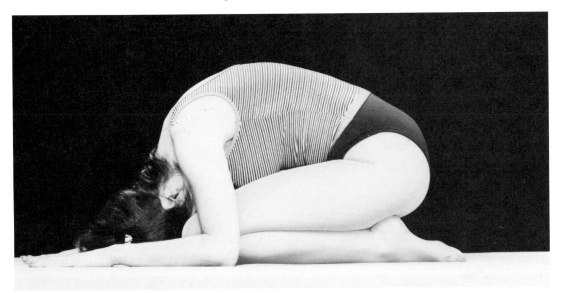

BENEFITS: Further stretches the muscles of the back. Muscles involved: Erector spinae, rhomboids, middle trapezius, buttocks and abdominal musculature.

POSTURE: Attempt to get your head to lie as close to your knees as possible.

CAUTION: Relax the head and neck.

SIDE-RELEASE STRETCH

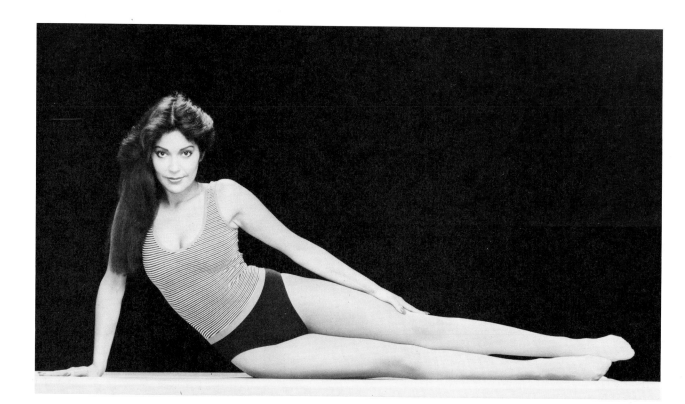

1 Roll to side with supporting arm straight.

2 Allow the trunk and pelvis to relax and feel the stretch along the outer abdominals and hip area.

3 Hold for eight counts.

4 Repeat on other side.

BENEFITS: Stretches the muscles that have been worked, and, if left unstretched, directly affect movement of the spine.
Muscles involved: Internal and external obliques as well as the quadratus lumborum and outer hip muscles, the gluteus medius, gluteus minimus and the tensor fasciae latae.

POSTURE: Keep the body in a straight line; support the arm directly below the shoulder. Keep the head and neck in a relaxed posture.

CAUTION: Don't allow tilting of the body in the back or front.

THE BARRE

Now for some fun!

You have just completed some very vigorous exercising. Now you have the opportunity to stretch and elongate those challenged muscles and, at the same time, feel like a dancer.

Not only should exercise improve the physical body, it should add enjoyment to the emotional part of living. This is one of the main reasons for the barre exercises.

The purpose of the barre movement is to stretch and lengthen the muscles in the back of the upper legs (hamstrings) and inner thighs (adductors).

When the leg is placed on the barre, that leg is no longer in a weight-bearing posture. Now the muscles are permitted to relax and stretch and elongate.

The barre exercises help you to develop a better sense of balance. There is also a sense of added grace and improved posture. You feel the same excitement a dancer feels.

So many people go through life thinking they are not graceful. They are sure they lack the ability to be a dancer. As they learn the movements at the barre, the confidence increases. Suddenly there is a new sense of self-esteem.

The barre will give you confidence.

You will be graceful.

You will move like a dancer.

THE EXERCISE

FLAT BACK/TRACTION STRETCH WITH PRESSURE ON/ PRESSURE OFF EXERCISE

1 Starting approximately arms distance from barre, grasp barre with the arms fully extended and allow your buttocks to drop back away from the barre. You should feel the traction stretch in the low back as you relax the entire trunk. Hold for eight counts.

2 Bring the body to erect position and gently allow the hips to lean forward toward the barre. Keep your buttocks and back muscles relaxed as the body extends forward.

3 Hold for eight counts.

BENEFITS: Stretches back, hamstrings and Achilles tendon during first part of exercise, and realigns the disc material in the second part of the exercise. Muscles involved: Back, hamstrings and Achilles tendon.

POSTURE: In position number 1, the head should be placed with ears next to arms. In both steps of the exercise the back muscles must remain relaxed.

HAMSTRING STRETCH

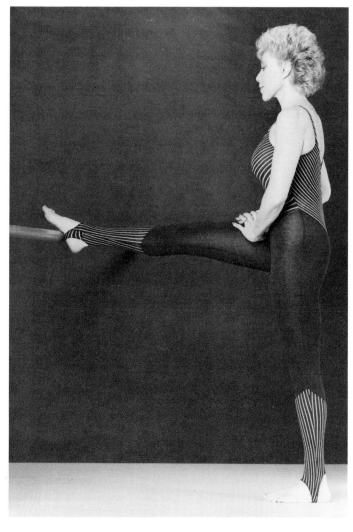
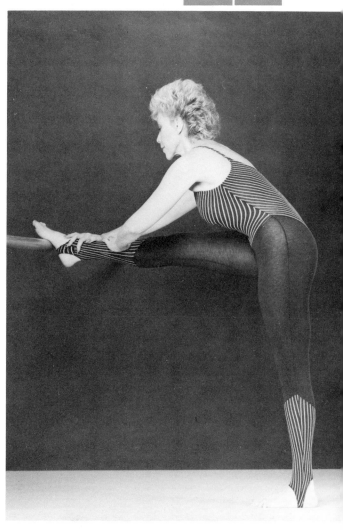

1 Stand a leg's distance from the barre. Place instep on the barre, keeping the foot flexed. Hips should be facing the barre.

2 While bending the upper body forward, slowly walk hands down the leg until you feel a stretch (no pain, but slight discomfort) throughout the back of the right leg.

3 Relax in the position for eight counts.

HAMSTRING STRETCH
CONTINUES
ON FOLLOWING PAGE

HAMSTRING STRETCH

4 Walk arms back up the legs to erect position (four counts).

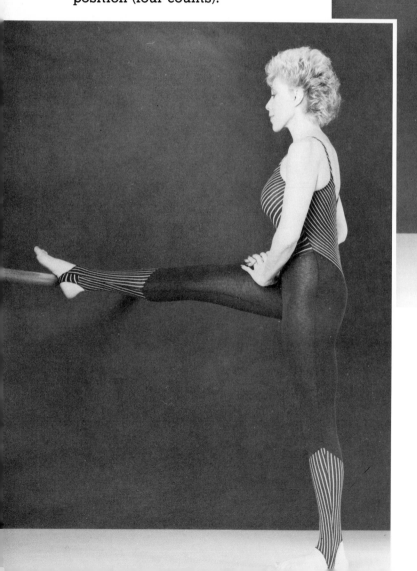

5 Place heel on the barre. Rotate the leg inward, keeping the hip and leg straight forward, and walk hands down the leg. Relax in position for eight counts; walk arms back up legs (four counts).

6 Rotate the leg outward and walk hands down the leg. Hold for eight counts; walk the arms back up the legs (four counts).

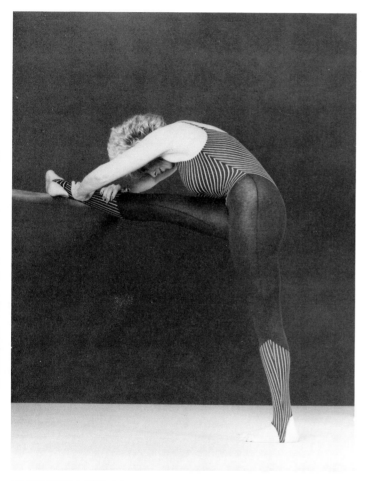
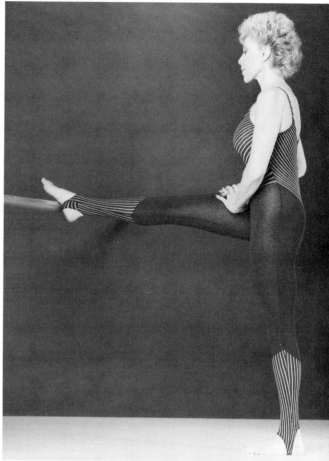

7 Return to starting position; repeat exercise on the other leg.

BENEFITS:	Stretches muscles in the leg (hamstrings). Stretches muscles commonly tight in the average person. Protects against spine injury by improving pelvic and spine mobility. Muscles involved: Inner and outer hamstrings.
POSTURE:	Keep hips relaxed.
CAUTION:	Don't permit the hip to lift. Do not enter painful stretch range.

THE EXERCISE
HIP FLEXOR STRETCH-UP

1 Place instep of foot on barre, with the leg bent.

2 While keeping standing leg straight, press supporting leg hip toward the barre for eight counts.

3 Slowly straighten the bent leg and hold for eight counts. Feel the stretch in the front of the hip of the weight-bearing leg.

4 Repeat on opposite side.

BENEFITS: Stretches the hip flexor muscle of the back leg and the upper hamstring and buttock muscle of the leg on the bar.
The hip flexor muscle if left unstretched pulls the spine forward, creating a dangerous swayback.
Muscles involved: Hamstring, buttocks and hip flexor.

POSTURE: Keep the heel of the standing leg flat on the floor.

CAUTION: Do not allow the back to arch.

THE EXERCISE
TAKE A BOW

WEEK 1 2 3 4

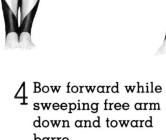

1 Stand sideways close to the barre.

2 Grasp the barre and lift free hand gracefully outward and over the head toward the barre. While leaning, bend sideways away from barre. Pull away for one count.

3 Return to vertical position and open free arm to the side.

4 Bow forward while sweeping free arm down and toward barre.

5 Return to upright position.

6 Repeat four times.

7 Repeat on other side.

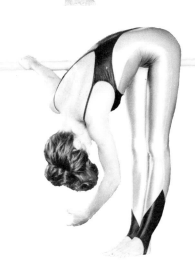

BENEFITS:	Stretches the entire side of body and releases tension. Protects the back by stretching the muscles that attach to the spine and rib cage. Muscles involved: Latissimus dorsi, quadratus lumborum and oblique abdominal muscles.
POSTURE:	Knees relaxed, abdominals tightened, chest up and chin pressed in.
CAUTION:	Keep feet together. Do not arch back.
MORE BENEFIT:	Increase range.

THE EXERCISE
QUADRICEP STRETCH

1 Stand sideways to the barre with feet together.

2 Lift heel toward buttocks and grasp the end of the foot.

3 Keeping the knees together, gently pull the foot toward buttocks . . . do not bend forward; do not arch the back.

4 Hold for four counts.

5 While still holding foot, relax position.

6 Repeat exercise four times.

7 Repeat exercise on other side.

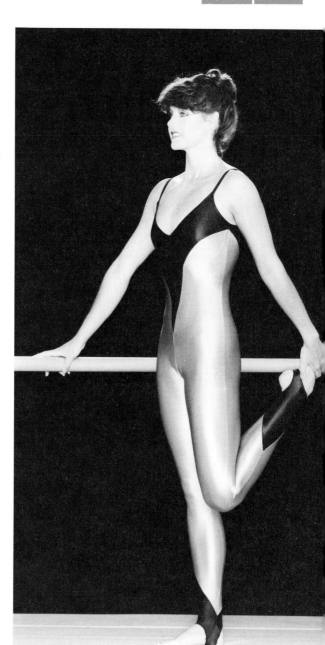

BENEFITS: Prevents formation of bulky muscles.
Stretches the strong muscles of the thigh and protects against common knee disorders.
Muscles involved: Quadriceps femoris.

POSTURE: Keep upper body lifted. Do not arch back.
Do not lean forward.

CAUTION: Maintain erect posture with chin in position.
Do not strain the shoulders.

THE COOL-DOWN

Ready for a rest?

The cool-down is one of the most important parts of the Body Design by Gilda exercise hour. It is so important that the body tissues you have just warmed cool slowly and that the muscles that have been so challenged in the last 60 minutes be permitted to readapt to a less demanding workload. This is the time you should relax your mind and body completely.

Here's how you cool down!

1. Lie flat on your back stretching out the body with the legs slightly apart, arms out to the sides with palms facing up. Eyes should be closed.
2. Inhale deeply through both nostrils. Then exhale. Repeat this deep breathing pattern four times.
3. Gently move the feet inward and outward, completely relaxing the muscles in the feet. Keep inhaling and exhaling. Let go of any tension that might be in your body.
4. Now move the entire leg inside, then outside. Keep relaxing and letting go of that tension. Keep breathing deeply.
5. Become aware of the abdomen. Inhale and exhale. Relax the muscles of the stomach area. Feel the muscles strengthening in the stomach. Now feel them relax.
6. Become aware of the muscles of the chest and breast area. Keep inhaling and exhaling. Notice the new feeling of vigor and warmth that has filled these muscles during the exercise hour.
7. Next become aware of the arms and shoulders. Stretch out the arms with the palms up and fingers relaxed. More deep breathing. Let those muscles relax.

8. Gently roll the head from side to side, letting go of the tension in the neck. Concentrating on the mouth, gently rotate the jaw around and around releasing all tension in that area. Sense the nose as the deep breathing continues. Gently tighten the eyelids. Open them and close them tightly. Now open them wide and close them, letting go of any tension in the brow and forehead.

9. Now for the final state of complete relaxation, close your mind from receiving all and any thoughts except the following countdown. As you go deep into relaxation, count: one and two and three and four . . . to a hundred. Concentrate deeply on the word "and" in between each number. Allow the body to completely relax and let go.

10. When you are ready to open your eyes after the hundred count, gently move the fingers, toes, feet, arms, hands. Open the eyes. Sense the reawakening of the energies of your body. Roll over onto your side in a prenatal position, pause a few moments, and very slowly sit up.

You will feel rejuvenated. You will feel relaxed. There will be an overall feeling of peace and tranquility. But most of all, you will have the desire and ability to meet the rest of the day's challenges with newfound energy and the satisfaction that you are alive and well.

CHAPTER 8
BE CAREFUL OF THAT BACK

*From the heart of this fountain of delight
wells up some bitter taste to choke them
even among the flowers.*

—LUCRETIUS

Throughout the Body Design by Gilda program, I have been alerting you to the dangers of hurting the back. This has become a serious problem. During the last decade, when physical fitness has become so much a part of everyone's life and well-being, a sad by-product of all this intense activity is—the bad back.

Seventy percent of all people will have one or more significant episodes of lower-back pain during their lives. Back pains account for more days off from work than any other illness. There are now many professionals and entire health industries that specifically treat low back pains: among them chiropractors, acupuncturists and therapeutic pain centers.

Most of the low-back pain injuries happen between the ages of thirty and fifty to people who are relatively sedentary, and most of these problems are caused by poor posture or strain.

Back pain can ruin an exercise program. The steady progress that has been made during the weeks and months of exercising can be halted by the period of inactivity often demanded by a flare-up of lower-back pain.

The Body Design by Gilda program has been carefully designed to avoid lower-back pain. While we stretch, we never overstretch. Look carefully at the photographs accompanying each exercise. They will show you exactly how far to stretch without straining. The idea is to coax the muscles, not to force them.

Exactly what is happening when the back hurts?

Every back ages. The cartilage of the bone wears away. The spine, a series of flexible joints, wears in its own natural pattern. If poor posture has caused this pattern to be slumped, the joints will wear prematurely. Also, between the joints, the spine has a kind of human shock absorber called discs; the discs have a tendency to compress in the front as gravity and poor posture make us slump forward.

Exercise can correct these problems.

Exercise can also make them worse.

Most of our lives we are slumped. As you read this chapter, check how you are sitting. Are you slumped in a sofa with your back curved? This habit causes the spine to naturally curve. Or are you propped up in bed with the neck and upper spine sharply curved? More of the same. You should be sitting with the lower back supported in its natural curve, preferably with a pillow under the low-back area to passively support the natural arching of this area of the spine. Sit back over the support and allow the chair to take some of the body weight off the discs. Both feet should be on the floor with the knees relaxed.

Now you realize that there is a good chance that you are coming into an exercise program with your back already damaged by years of poor posture habits. What happens? Without proper and careful warm-up, you try to force that less-than-perfect spine into motions designed for a perfect spine. Sometimes under the misguided notion that overpushing the range of an exercise increases the benefit (Wrong!), you extend the scope of the exercise.

And something snaps.

Exercise is really the least of the culprits that cause the bad back. Our day-to-day life-styles cause far more problems than even improperly done exercise.

Suppose you have spent ten minutes bent over looking into the lower drawer of a file cabinet. The pressure is directly on the front of the spine. All the fluids inside the shock-absorber discs have moved backward. Then you stand up quickly. The ligaments holding the fluid inside the disc tear and the fluid ruptures. This is a slipped disc.

The one certain way to avoid this type of injury is to keep the back muscles, tendons and ligaments exercised and limber. In addition, you need to practice good posture and offset all of the forward flexion present in our daily life-styles with passive backward extension.

Start improving your posture—now!

1. Sit straight in a chair, with feet resting on the ground.
2. When you are sitting, use a backrest to keep the back slightly arched with back supports (perhaps a pillow). This is

especially important while driving. Don't strain forward in the car seat. Sit back and give the neck support and enjoy the ride.

3. Don't lean forward while you are sitting. This is one of the most potentially damaging positions for the back. Sit back and let the seat back take some weight off your spine.

4. Using a typewriter places even more pressures on the discs and spine than writing by hand at a desk. The height of the typewriter should be adjusted downward. It is a good idea to stand and stretch frequently while typing. Keep desk and typewriter close to your stomach. This will keep you from leaning forward. Your back will be supported better in this position.

5. That slightly bent position that is so common while making beds, using the sweeper, washing, scrubbing and cooking is very bad for the back. Try to eliminate this position completely. This can be achieved by raising the heights of the work areas (higher shelves) or adjusting the work tools (a taller sweeper handle), or hiring a maid. If work must be done on the floor, it is more comfortable and better posture to be on all fours so long as the back is not permitted to sag.

6. Lifting anything should be avoided as much as possible. If it is necessary to lift something, avoid bending or flexing the back. Instead, bend the knees while keeping the spine as straight as possible with whatever is being lifted held close to the body.

7. Avoid overextending the spine while sleeping. Do not lay flat on your stomach in a prone position. If you prefer sleeping in a prone position, place a pillow under the stomach or side to give the spine a slight tilt.

Whether exercising or just participating in everyday life, you should become aware of the need to balance the demands of the back. This means that when you spend time bent forward you should also make it a habit to bend backward to release the muscles and ligaments and to recenter the fluid that makes up the inside of the discs. Throughout the day you should passively, and with care, bend backward or arch the back to achieve an overall balance of the spine.

The standing pressure-on/pressure-off maneuver is done with the feet spread at shoulder width, and the hands placed on the buttocks or in the small of the back. Now simply push forward with your hands, allowing the back to passively arch over your hands. The back and buttock muscles must remain relaxed.

Bend to the end of your available range of motion in this direction. Do not stop in the fully arched position. Once you've reached the end, simply let off the pressure and allow the spine to return to a straight position. Repeat five to ten times throughout the day—especially before and after any forward bending or sitting activity.

Another great exercise to ease the strain on the back is a "passive push-up." This is done by laying on your stomach, flat on the floor, and just raising the upper body with the arms. Feel the back stretch into place. Keep the pelvis on the floor and the back and buttock muscles relaxed. There goes the tension out of the back. The only muscles being forced into use should be the muscles in the arms.

The more you do this exercise . . . the better the back will be.

This does not mean that by following these exercises you can correct a damaged back. A damaged back requires professional help. The above exercises should not cause pain. There may be some discomfort in the low back, especially at first, as you enter a range of motion probably not used in a long while. If the discomfort is only present in the "up" position, and goes away as you let the pressure off, and does not increase with each repetition but improves, then you are doing the back some good.

On the other hand, if pain is experienced with each pressure on movement and it increases with each repetition or radiates out of the back and into the leg, then you need professional help from a physical therapist or a doctor.

But by watching your posture, stretching, and being aware of your back, you can keep it in the best possible condition. And by following a carefully planned exercise program, you can correct the damage that has become a part of today's confused life-style that has a person sitting at a desk part of a day and then straining to run miles on hard concrete.

It is sad that many people are unaware of what all this poor posture is doing to the quality of their lives. They become used to the slight pain in the back. It is only when something serious happens to intensify that pain that most people decide to be more careful of the back. A fit person, on the other hand, leads a far more effortless life. A life without back pains. A life where the back functions easily.

A Gilda Rule: Try Not to Bend That Back. Bend the Knees and Stretch Those Arms Instead.

The possibility of damaging the back is present in athletic activities, but with careful preparation through exercise, serious injuries can be avoided. The posture you assume after athletics is often more damaging than the sport itself. As the muscles cool down and naturally tighten a bit, we often find ourselves slouched over a bar stool sipping beverages, or plopped in an overstuffed sofa.

The muscles tighten in terrible postures and afterward, movement is painful, tight and damaging. Proper posture is a must after athletic movements. Sit with your back supported and give your body a chance to recuperate in good alignment.

Remember to stretch those muscles. Remember to counteract all that slumping with extension and stretching exercise.

Remember to warm up that back.

Remember to properly cool down the back after vigorously exercising it.

And most important . . . remember to be *aware* of the back.

CHAPTER 9
THE ALL-DAY WORKOUT

Make your life into an exercise program!

One of the reasons a person gets out-of-shape is over the years he abandons exercising. Children are always exercising. They seem to be running and playing all day long. But as we become adults, we find reasons for not exercising. It is then that a person really needs to start a planned exercise program. Reasons such as: I don't have time. I'm too tired.

None of these reasons are valid. Saying you don't have time to exercise is an excuse. I actively manage two businesses, have a family, and never stop exercising. Some of the important businesspeople and celebrities who come to my studio have tremendous demands filling every moment of their days, but always make the time to exercise. They look at exercise as an obligation they owe themselves. The exercise helps them to relax and at the same time gives them increased physical strength to continue their high-pressured daily lives.

A Gilda Rule: Use Your Body Every Minute of Every Day.

Start by learning to walk again.

I usually walk several miles every morning with a certain portion of this hiking going up and down hills. This helps to increase the cardiovascular benefits of walking. I walk at a brisk pace, being careful to take deep breaths through the nose and breathe out through the mouth.

Walking has become an important part of my fitness discipline.

If I have an appointment within walking distance, I leave the car in the garage and walk. I walk to lunch. If I feel tense or ill-tempered at the end of the day, I walk. Through walking I not only improve my physical condition but add the all-so-necessary quiet time to my life to calm and organize me mentally. At night, instead of watching television, I walk and think about the day I have completed and the plans for the following day. I use walking as an exercise reward instead of an exercise obligation. *Exercise should be a reward.*

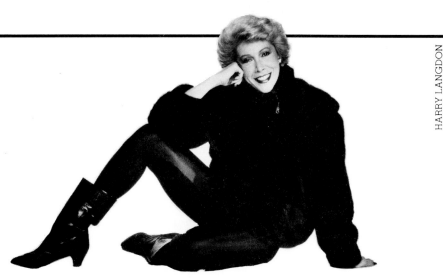

But there are more ways to make exercise a part of your day. Often I have heard people complain that they were never out-of-shape until they went to work behind a desk. The office is blamed for many a protruding stomach and spreading derriere. This is really a flabby excuse.

The office job does not have to doom a person to a future of sagging muscles and a bulging waistline. Exercise can be a part of the office routine. Every movement can be an exercise, even while sitting behind a desk. It is not necessary to leave the office to exercise. It is not necessary to put on a track suit and run laps during the lunch hour (although if you like to do this, it is fine). But it is necessary to reorganize the daily office routine to include beneficial movement.

Office routine can be damaging to your body.

Sitting in a chair for hours will weaken the back muscles, especially if you are sitting in a chair without arms and permit your body to slump. Typing is particularly hard on the posture, as the arms and hands are in an unnatural position placing strain on the back and shoulders. Slumping forward will weaken the stomach muscles. All this helps to cause what has been dubbed the middle-age spread.

But even long periods of sitting can be beneficial. Just learn to sit correctly.

Select a sturdy chair. Avoid a chair that tilts. All legs of the chair should be on the floor. Place both feet (yours, not the chair's) firmly on the floor and slightly spread apart. Hold on to the sides of the chair (not the arms but under the seat). Sit erect and concentrate on pulling in the stomach muscles. Don't permit anything to sag. Elongate the spine. Stretch upward—hold in those stomach muscles. Hold it in for the count of five. Then relax. Keep breathing . . . *Do not hold your breath during the five-count.* This exercise can be done anytime, anywhere—even while you are stuck in the rush hour traffic in your automobile.

That was an easy one, wasn't it?

Next, sit back in the chair, and again grasp the bottom of the seat. Place the feet shoulder width apart. Pull in the stomach muscles. Lift the legs straight out in front . . . if you can. This is challenging, but it does wonderful things for the legs. Hold those legs out there for several seconds, then lower them very slowly. This will exercise and stretch many of the leg muscles. Be sure to protect the back by not permitting it to arch during this exercise.

The neck and shoulders are another area that get very tight when not exercised regularly. Office pressures and tensions also seem to affect these areas first. To release tension in the neck and shoulders, sit straight in the chair. Clasp your hands behind your neck with the elbows slightly forward. Press the hands forward as you press the head backward. The tension and knotted muscles seem to disappear.

All relaxed now?

A reverse of this exercise is to clasp your hands on your forehead (again with the elbows out) and press the head forward while pushing back with the palms of your hands. Make the pressure smooth and controlled. Avoid jarring motions.

To loosen the neck and back while sitting, tilt your head toward your shoulder and roll the head slowly around front to the other shoulder. Reverse the direction and repeat several times.

Here is a more difficult exercise.

Again, while sitting in a chair, place both feet on the floor. Lean forward and grasp the ankles. Pretend you have dropped a pencil under the desk and you are looking for it. Then, while still holding the ankles, flatten out the back into a straight (or as straight as possible) line.

Even the file cabinet can be transformed into a piece of exercise equipment. Stand facing the file cabinet. Hold on to the sides. Do "outside leg lifts." Keeping the knee straight, lift the leg straight out to the side. This might look silly, but it is wonderful for the legs and hips. Think of the barre movements. This is an opportunity to do some light exercise during the office day.

There is the wall press for calf stretching. Place both palms against the wall at shoulder level, with the feet approximately three feet from the wall and at hip distance apart. Bend the elbows so the body moves closer to the wall, keeping the back and legs in a straight line. Feel the stretch in the calf area. Keep the heels on the floor.

Sit down again.

This has been dubbed the alphabet exercise. While sitting with the legs crossed, work the ankles and toes by writing out an imaginary alphabet with the foot. This can be a psychological as well as a physical exercise. One person I know has progressed past merely writing the alphabet and has started writing out words and opinions that only she knows. Do not tell your boss about this emotional release or he (or she) might start reading your feet!

All of these exercises should become a comfortable part of your daily routine. And if they are performed every day (as many times as you want), it will not be long until your physical and mental capacities are vastly improved.

Some of you might be thinking that it would be either embarrassing or impossible to do these exercises at your office. Maybe the boss wouldn't approve of you using the file cabinet as a barre. Maybe you might feel self-conscious jiggling around a desk chair.

Don't! Don't be hesitant to improve your health.

Make exercising into an office project. Get co-workers to join you. Exchange that coffee and danish break for a five-minute exercise session.

A fit person makes good business sense.

CHAPTER 10
A LAST WORD FROM GILDA

It's a lot of effort!

The Body Design by Gilda program requires that you devote at least three hours each week to performing a carefully choreographed and challenging exercise program. The program needs the support of individual self-discipline; the self-discipline to avoid overeating and binging, the self-discipline to always keep the body properly rested, and the self-discipline to make the program an important part of your life.

Your life can be so wonderful.

Mine is.

The program is a wonderful cycle. You exercise and get stronger. As you get stronger you have more energy to exercise and enjoy your life. And the brain is constantly being fed with oxygen. You feel more alert because you are more alert. Just as the muscles have been toned and stimulated, so has the brain.

The Body Design by Gilda program cannot be treated as the latest of a never-ending series of books that are bought, read, followed for a while, and forgotten. It is a wonderful way of life. It is a way of life I want you to have.

A lot of the rich and famous people of the world have naturally gravitated to my exercise studio in Beverly Hills, people such as Marlo Thomas (she exercises to give her the energy for her very involved life) and Britt Ekland (she always has some handsome young hunk waiting for her after class). Britt admits that the Body Design by Gilda program has become a very important part of her life. "Oh, I had exercised before," she said one day after class while some great-looking guy paced in the lobby, "but with your method, things just changed." She does the program daily because her body is an important part of her career and her future. "Although I find the aerobics so challenging, I'll keep coming back until I'm too old, frail, sick or whatever. At forty (she looks twenty), I am proud to be a fit student of yours." Britt Ekland has made the Body Design by Gilda her workout.

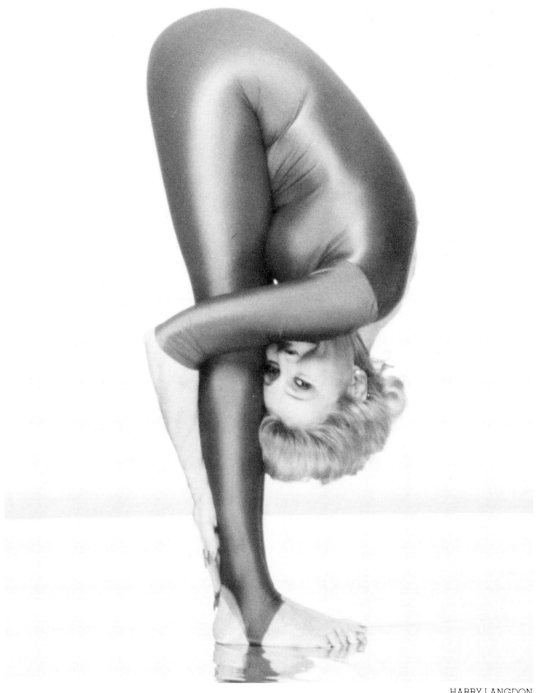

HARRY LANGDON

207 A LAST WORD FROM GILDA

Singer Marilyn McCoo also does the program daily although because of travel, she must usually do it in a hotel room someplace. "I have firmed, toned and reshaped my body with no unsightly muscular development," she explained. "That's for me!"

There have been many people helped by the Body Design by Gilda program who do not have famous names. People who have pride in themselves. People who want to look and feel better. People who are willing to put a little effort into making their lives better.

You can make your life better too!

Even your sex life should improve.

I am reminded of my own honeymoon. When I married Bob we decided to honeymoon in Hawaii. I always tell the hotel reservations people I want a room large enough for exercising and this time we got the honeymoon suite. Bob was still getting used to my passion for exercising and enthusiastically participated in my daily exercise routine.

Now, when I exercise with my students or my husband, I yell encouragement. Inside the honeymoon suite, I was yelling to be heard over the disco music (remember, always use music when exercising).

And my voice was carrying.

"Get it up . . . come on . . . you can get it up more."

"Push . . . one . . . two . . . three . . . four."

"You can do it!"

"More . . . more . . . MORE!"

While I was inspiring my husband to put more effort into exercising, the hallway outside the honeymoon suite became a gathering place for the curious. When we opened the doors there was a group of interested faces wanting to see this couple who sounded so eager in the honeymoon suite. I have since learned to regulate my voice while exercising in hotels.

Sex has sometimes been called an athletic event, and a good part of it is. Great sex (like any physically demanding activity) requires that the people participating be flexible, energetic and enthusiastic. But more important, people need to feel positive and more secure about themselves. This helps them to be more imaginative and creative. They have the necessary endurance to really experience sex.

Most of my students did not originally come to my classes to improve their sex lives, but as their conditions and physical appearances improved, that is exactly

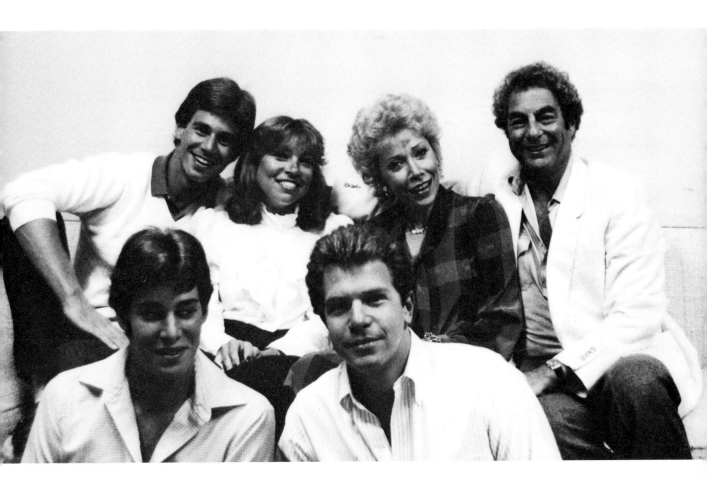

what happened. Exercise improves the sexual appetite. This has caused drastic changes in some of my women students' marital lives. As their bodies start to improve, their need and enthusiasm for sex also increases.

It is not unusual for a woman to come to me after a workout and say, "I have noticed a change in my life! The problem areas in the relationship with my husband have improved." What she means is they are making love better and more frequently.

Some women frankly admit, "I like making love longer and more often," while others simply remark, "I feel young again."

Usually, husbands are very enthusiastic about their wives' increased enthusiasm for sex, but there are exceptions. I remember one woman who had done a fabulous job of resculpturing herself and had lots of energy for—everything. Unfortunately, her husband didn't. "I had better get my husband into some kind of exercise program or get another husband," she said. He didn't! And she did!

In my exercise studios I keep a notebook where my students are encouraged to write their comments. So often their words are eloquent and touching: "This has changed my life . . . I am so happy with myself . . . my husband never wants me to stop the program . . . I know I am somebody now." These are all the words of the encouraged. Even though not all of these people might have resculptured themselves into the images they hoped for when starting the program, they are all success stories. They all feel better about themselves. More energy and excitement has been added to the quality of their lives.

We all need to feel encouraged. That is so important.

I am so grateful for the encouragement I have received. As I reread those comment books from my studios (I do this frequently), I am so glad to have had the opportunity to give hope and encouragement to thousands of people. It was this kind of encouragement that convinced me to write this book so that perhaps millions of persons can feel the way I feel. I want to encourage you just as that wonderful man so many years ago encouraged the fat little girl dancing her heart out on a little Pittsburgh recital stage:

"Say . . . she is great!"

My life has changed so much since I have had the physical and mental energy to meet it head-on. So many wonderful things have happened to me because I was not too tired or too beaten to take a chance at opportunity.

I know what is important in my life and it starts with being physically and mentally able to attack life enthusiastically every day. My life is very filled with activity. There never seems to be enough hours in the day. The days are only short because I want to fill every moment with something rewarding.

I wake up turned-on. My life is very full. I am always taking on a new project to utilize all the energy that is now a part of me. I always have six balls in the air. Sometimes those balls bump into each other but when that happens I have the strength to pick them up and toss them into the air again.

Both my husband Bob and I know what it means to have the energy to start over. When we married ten years ago, we had both had two divorces and business difficulties (and successes). We are both high-energy people. Our talents and enthusiasms (he is the business head of our nine corporations and I do the creating) are constantly complementing each other. We have the strength to understand, support and inspire one another.

My husband and my children are the most important people in my life. Our eldest son, Greg Marx, is a successful actor in the soap opera *Days of Our Lives*. Daughter, Laura Lynn, has started her career in the fashion retail business. Mitchell has joined us in the family business (Flexatard, Inc.). Christopher is building robots at ITT and Tracy attends Michigan State University.

In spite of a demanding business schedule, I have the energy to enjoy, spending time with my family, my mother, Ruth, sister June and brothers Dave and Leonard, and their families nearby.

The foundation of my life is the Body Design by Gilda program. It gives me the physical and mental strength to be what I should be. Without feeling great, I wouldn't be at peg one.

I am so very grateful for my life. I think I have it all. A man respects and loves me. My children are happy. I have success. I have a beautiful home. But the key to it all is I have a philosophy that keeps me strong and eager to create my world. It all starts with having the strength and will to live a wonderful life.

The Body Design by Gilda program and philosophy worked for me. I have seen it work for others. Please, let it work for you.

Have the energy.

Have a wonderful life!

GILDA MARX

GLOSSARY

ABDOMINAL MUSCLES—these muscles make up the front and side walls of the trunk from the bottom of the ribs to the pelvis. They function to support the organs and perform a curling of the upper trunk or rib cage, shoulders, and head on the pelvis. They also assist in a twisting of the trunk on the pelvis. They include the rectus abdominis and the internal and external oblique muscles.

AEROBIC EXERCISE—exercise performed continuously for a period of time and at an intensity high enough to increase the heart rate to at least 85 percent of its maximum rate.

ANAEROBIC EXERCISE—exercise performed at very high levels of intensity that cannot be sustained for very long.

BALLISTIC MOVEMENT—uncontrolled body movements.

BICEPS—a two-headed muscle located on the top of the arm between the shoulder and the elbow.

CALORIE—a unit of heat; the amount of heat required to raise the temperature of one gram of water one degree Centigrade, or a unit for measuring the heat value of food.

CARBOHYDRATE—an organic compound; includes starches, sugars and cellulose.

CELLULOSE—a fibrous carbohydrate that is the main structural component of plant tissue.

CONNECTIVE TISSUE—tough, fibrous tissue that makes up the framework of muscle, ligaments, tendons and fasciae.

COOL-DOWN—the time needed to bring the body back to the original energy level. To cool the body, slow down the heart rate.

DEHYDRATION—the condition that results from undue water loss.

DELTOID—a three-part muscle that forms a cap over the shoulder and is largely responsible for movements of the shoulder.

DISC—the cartilage shock absorbers found between the bones of the spine called vertebrae.

ENDORPHINS—the opiate-like chemicals produced naturally in the brain and released in response to stress to the body, such as exercise. They act to reduce perception of pain and may act as a mood elevator.

ENDURANCE—performance duration.

ENERGY—the capacity to do work.

ERECTOR SPINAE—the lower back muscles found in the small of the back, they perform an arching of the bones of the lower spine. They also act to stabilize the pelvis so the thigh bones can move on a stationary base.

FAT—oily or greasy matter making up the bulk of adipose tissue.

FIRM—compressed hardness; compact and dense.

FLEX—to move muscles so as to cause flexion of a joint.

FLEXIBILITY—that property of muscles and connective tissue which allows for full range of motion.

FLEXION—movement that decreases the angle at a joint; the act of bending the joint.

GLUCOSE—the simplest form of sugar in which a carbohydrate is assimilated in the body; blood sugar.

GLUTEUS MAXIMUS, MEDIUS AND MINIMUS—the three muscles that give shape to the buttocks and serve as powerful mobilizers of the hip joint.

GOOD POSTURE—alignment of the body parts so that a plumb line would intersect the earlobe, shoulder, hip, knee and ankle.

HAMSTRINGS—the three muscles that make up the bulk of the back of the thigh are the biceps femoris, semimembranosus and the semitendinosus. They act at the knee to cause further bending of the thigh backward from the body.

HEART RATE—the frequency of the contractions of the heart usually reported in beats per minute.

HIP ABDUCTORS—the muscles making up the bulk of the side of the buttocks. They enable the thigh to move away from the body. These muscles include the gluteus medius, gluteus minimus and the tensor fasciae latae.

HIP ADDUCTORS—the muscles that make up the bulk of the inner thigh which enable the thigh to cross the midline of the body. They include the adductor magnus, adductor longus, adductor brevis and the gracilis.

HIP FLEXORS—although many muscles assist in the forward movement of the thigh, the prime movers are the iliacus and psoas muscles (iliopsoas group).

HYPEREXTENSION—extension of a body segment past the anatomical position.

INTERVERTEBRAL DISC—the discs of the fibrocartilage between bodies of vertebrae.

INTRAMUSCULAR FAT—marble fat within the muscle.

ISOMETRIC CONTRACTION—a contraction in which the muscle tension increases, but the muscle does not shorten because it does not overcome the resistance.

ISOTONIC CONTRACTION—a contraction in which muscle fibers change length as a result of stimulus.

JOINT CAPSULE—a sac-like structure of connective tissue that encapsulates a joint.

LATERAL—away from the midline of the body.

LEAN BODY MASS—the mass of the body minus the fat, which leaves bone, muscle and connective tissue.

LIGAMENTS—tough fibrous tissue that connects one bone to another.

LUNGE—to plunge forward.

MAXIMUM HEART RATE—the maximum frequency of heart contractions possible per minute.

METABOLIC RATE—the energy expended by the body per unit of time.

METABOLISM—the sum total of the chemical reactions that occur within the body.

METABOLIZE—the chemical change in living cells by which energy is produced and new material is assimilated for the repair and replacement of tissue.

MUSCLE—the motors of the body that create movement by contracting; responsible for bodily strength.

MUSCLE CONTRACTION—the development of tension within a muscle that can cause a joint to move.

MUSCULAR STRENGTH—strength is the force that a muscle, or muscle group can exert in one maximal contraction.

NUTRIENT—a substance needed by a living thing to maintain life, health and reproduction.

OBLIQUES—abdominal muscles located on the sides of the middle abdomen.

OVERLOAD—doing a little bit more than you did before; increasing the intensity of an exercise, increasing the duration.

PECTORALS—the large fan-shaped muscles that occupy the area over the upper ribs known as the chest. These muscles move the arm across the midline of the body as well as performing pushing and hugging type movements.

PELVIS—the bony skeleton making up the lower trunk and hips.

PLUMB LINE—a line dropped from the ceiling with a weight on the bottom used for evaluation of upright standing posture. The line represents the direction of the forces of gravity.

PROPER BODY ALIGNMENT—body segments must be aligned one on top of the other to achieve body balance and proper posture.

PROTEIN—the major source of building tissue for muscles, blood, skin, hair, nails and internal organs including the heart.

QUADRATUS LUMBORUM—a muscle found in the area of the low back extending from the lower ribs to the pelvis posteriorly. The action of this muscle is to elevate or hike the hip.

QUADRICEPS—four muscles located on the top of the thigh; the rectus femoris, vastus intermedius, vastus lateralis and the vastus medialis.

QUADRICEPS FEMORIS—a group of four muscles on the front of the thigh that act to straighten the knee joint.

RECTUS ABDOMINIS—the abdominal muscle which runs down the center of the body from the rib cage to the pubis.

RELAXATION—releasing unwanted muscular tension within the body.

RESTING HEART RATE—the frequency of the contractions of the heart per minute when at rest.

RHOMBOIDS—the muscles located in between the shoulder blades that are responsible for stabilizing and rotating the shoulder blades.

SKELETAL MUSCLE—the muscles responsible for the movement of bones.

SQUAT—to settle down as if sitting or crouching.

STATIC STRETCHING—holding a muscle on a sustained stretch to allow a relaxation of the muscle and achieve the best benefits.

STRENGTHENING EXERCISE—exercise performed against some form of resistance that leads to strengthening of the muscles responsible for that particular movement.

STRETCHING EXERCISE—any movement that lengthens structures such as muscles, fasciae, ligaments and tendons.

SUBCUTANEOUS FAT—fat deposited under the skin and over the muscles.

TARGET HEART RATE—the rate at which you want to raise your pulse to achieve a maximum training effect.

TENDONS—the connective tissue structures that make up the part of the muscle which attaches to a bone.

TRAINING HEART RATE—the frequency of the heart rate per minute during aerobic exercise.

TRAPEZIUS—the muscle located at the base of the neck that runs to the top of the shoulder.

TRICEPS—the three-headed muscle located on the back of the arm between the shoulder and the elbow.

VERTEBRAE—the bony segments of the spine.

VITAMINS—organic substances found in foods which perform specific and vital functions in the cells and tissues of the body.

WARM-UP—the process of gradually stretching the major muscle groups with mild exercise to literally warm up the body or to create body heat.

BODY CHART I

ANTERIOR VIEW

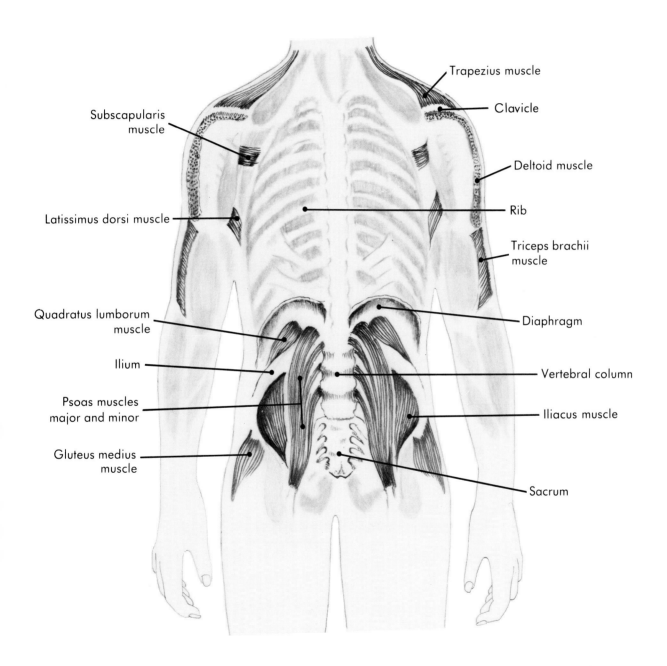

Subscapularis muscle

Latissimus dorsi muscle

Quadratus lumborum muscle

Ilium

Psoas muscles major and minor

Gluteus medius muscle

Trapezius muscle

Clavicle

Deltoid muscle

Rib

Triceps brachii muscle

Diaphragm

Vertebral column

Iliacus muscle

Sacrum

BODY CHART II

ANTERIOR VIEW

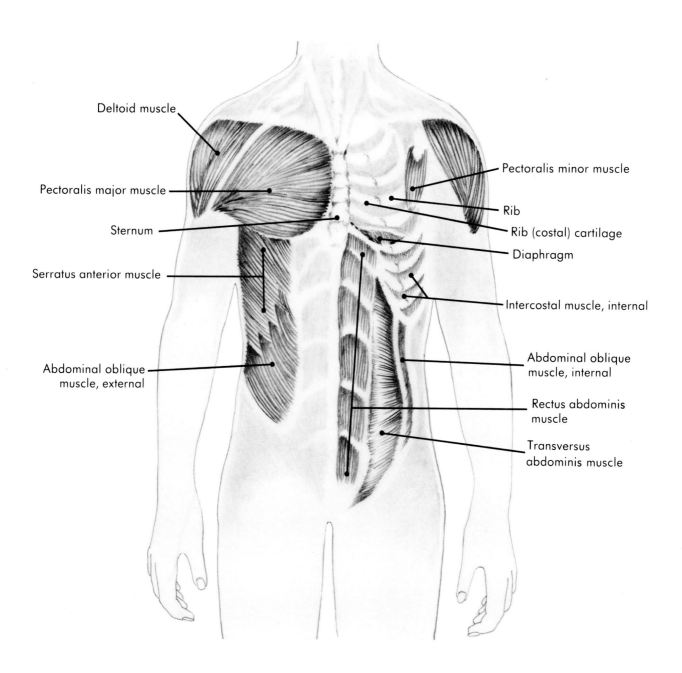

Deltoid muscle

Pectoralis major muscle

Sternum

Serratus anterior muscle

Abdominal oblique
muscle, external

Pectoralis minor muscle

Rib

Rib (costal) cartilage

Diaphragm

Intercostal muscle, internal

Abdominal oblique
muscle, internal

Rectus abdominis
muscle

Transversus
abdominis muscle

BODY CHART III

POSTERIOR VIEW

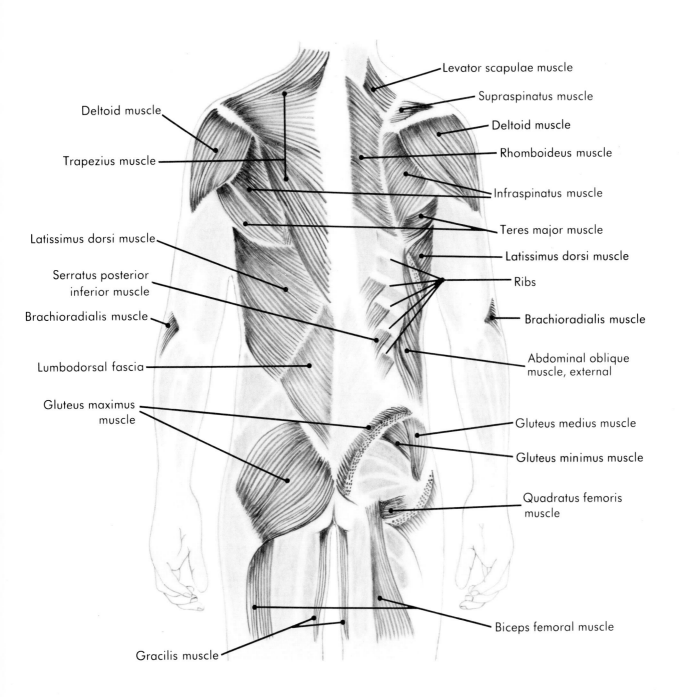

Deltoid muscle

Trapezius muscle

Latissimus dorsi muscle

Serratus posterior inferior muscle

Brachioradialis muscle

Lumbodorsal fascia

Gluteus maximus muscle

Gracilis muscle

Levator scapulae muscle

Supraspinatus muscle

Deltoid muscle

Rhomboideus muscle

Infraspinatus muscle

Teres major muscle

Latissimus dorsi muscle

Ribs

Brachioradialis muscle

Abdominal oblique muscle, external

Gluteus medius muscle

Gluteus minimus muscle

Quadratus femoris muscle

Biceps femoral muscle

BODY DESIGN BY GILDA STUDIOS

BEACHWOOD, OHIO (CLEVELAND)

Pavilion Mall
24075 Chagrin Blvd.
Beachwood, Ohio 44122
216/821-5023

DALLAS, TEXAS

220 Preston Valley Shopping Center
Dallas, Texas 75230
214/788-1822

HOUSTON, TEXAS

12520 Memorial Drive
Houston, Texas 77024
713/465-2950

LA JOLLA, CALIFORNIA

926 Turquoise Center
La Jolla, California 92109
619/483-5060

LOS ANGELES, CALIFORNIA (CENTURY CITY)

2080 Century Park East, Penthouse
Los Angeles, California 90067
213/553-2512

MANHASSET, NEW YORK

1482 Northern Blvd.
Manhasset, New York 11030
516/365-6220

NEW YORK, NEW YORK

1407 Broadway
New York, New York 10018
212/398-1407

NEW YORK, NEW YORK

139 East 57th Street
New York, New York 10022
212/759-7966

NEW YORK, NEW YORK

187 East 79th Street
New York, New York 10021
212/737-8440

NEW YORK, NEW YORK

65 W. 70th Street (At Columbus Ave.)
New York, New York 10023
212/799-8540

STAMFORD, CONNECTICUT

2329 Summer Street
Stamford, Connecticut 06905
203/324-BODY

TORONTO, ONTARIO (CANADA)

1290 Bay Street
Toronto, Ontario, Canada
416/928-0737

WASHINGTON, D.C.

4801 Wisconsin Avenue NW
Washington, D.C. 20016
202/363-4801

Audio and videotapes of the
Body Design by Gilda
program will be available soon.
For information about the tapes,
please write to:

Gilda Marx
Tape Department
1755 Exposition Boulevard
Los Angeles, California 90064